Magnetic Resonance Imaging

STUDY GUIDE AND EXAM REVIEW

Magnetic Resonance Imaging

STUDY GUIDE AND EXAM REVIEW

Stewart C. Bushong, Sc.D., FACR, FACMP
Professor of Radiologic Science
Baylor College of Medicine
Houston, Texas

with 201 illustrations

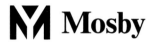

St. Louis Baltimore Boston Carlsbad Chicago Naples New York Philadelphia Portland
London Madrid Mexico City Singapore Sydney Tokyo Toronto Wiesbaden

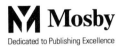
Mosby
Dedicated to Publishing Excellence

A Times Mirror
Company

Editor: Jeanne Rowland
Developmental Editor: Lisa Potts
Design and Layout: Winnie Sullivan
Project Manager: Gayle Morris
Manufacturing Supervisor: Betty Richmond

FIRST EDITION

Printed in the United States of America

Mosby-Year Book, Inc.
11830 Westline Industrial Drive
St. Louis, Missouri 63146

Library of Congress Cataloging-in-Publication Data

ISBN 0-8151-1340-4

96 97 98 99 00 / 9 8 7 6 5 4 3 2 1

To:

Bettie,
Leslie,
Stephen,
Andrew,
Butterscotch, †
Jemimah, †
Geraldine, †
Casper, †
Ginger, †
Sebastian, †
Buffy, †
Brie, †
Linus, †
Midnight, †
Boef, †
Cassie, †
Lucy, †
Toto, †
Molly, †
Ebony, †
Cody, †
Chandon
Meisha
Tuppence

† R.I.P.

❒ PREFACE

This study guide is designed to support the technologist and radiologist in preparing for their respective credentialing examinations. The organization is keyed to the companion textbook Magnetic Resonance Imaging: Physical and Biological Principles, where answers to each of these study questions will be found.

The organization of this study guide is also in keeping with the categories of content specifications for the ARRT examination in Magnetic Resonance Imaging. The worksheets that apply to each of the content categories are as follows:

Content Category

A. Physical Principles of Image Formation:
   Worksheets Number 1-32

B. Data Acquisition and Processing:
   Worksheets Number 33-44

C. Imaging Procedures:
   Worksheets Number 45-68

D. Patient Care and MRI Safety:
   Worksheets Number 69-75

I'm deeply grateful to my friend and fellow Texan, LuAnn Culbreath, at Baylor University Medical Center in Dallas, for providing the section on imaging procedures—Worksheets Number 45-68, including all of the images.

I am also grateful to Rodney Roemer of Triton College, Illinois, for the suggestion of adding the *Questions To Ponder* at the end of each worksheet. Many of these *QTPs* were contributed by Mr. Roemer, and I believe they represent a significant addition to each worksheet.

Many thanks also to Judy Matteau Faldyn for her attention and diligence in the preparation of this manuscript.

I have tried to structure the information in this study guide at a level of difficulty somewhat higher than that which I expect of the ARRT examination. I feel confident that if students of this study guide can answer questions of this level of difficulty, they will do exceptionally well on their respective examinations. I would appreciate any feedback from technologists who have taken the ARRT examination regarding how close this study guide meets its goals.

If we continue to communicate and exchange information we'll reach the goal that we all share of making physics fun.

Stewart C. Bushong

☐ TABLE OF CONTENTS

SECTION I
PHYSICAL PRINCIPLES OF IMAGE FORMATION

Part One   **Introduction**

Worksheet 1   Historical Trail, 3
Worksheet 2   Why do MRI?, 5
Worksheet 3   MRI Briefly, 7
Worksheet 4   Electrostatics, 11

Part Two   **Instrumentation**

Worksheet 5   Electrodynamics, 13
Worksheet 6   Magnetism, 15
Worksheet 7   Electromagnetism, 17
Worksheet 8   Electromagnetic Radiation, 19
Worksheet 9   The Gantry/Operating Console, 23
Worksheet 10   Primary Magnets, 27
Worksheet 11   Shim Coils, 29
Worksheet 12   Gradient Coils, 31
Worksheet 13   The RF Probe, 35
Worksheet 14   Selecting the Imager, 37
Worksheet 15   Locating the Imager, 39
Worksheet 16   Designing the Facility, 41
Worksheet 17   Quantum Mechanical Description, 43

Part Three   **Fundamentals**

Worksheet 18   Classical Mechanical Description, 47
Worksheet 19   Net Magnetization, 49
Worksheet 20   Reference Frames, 51
Worksheet 21   RF Pulses, 53
Worksheet 22   Spin Density, 57
Worksheet 23   T1 Relaxation Time, 59
Worksheet 24   T2 Relaxation Time, 61
Worksheet 25   How to Measure T2, 63
Worksheet 26   How to Measure T1, 65
Worksheet 27   Nuclear Species, 67
Worksheet 28   Chemical Shift, 69
Worksheet 29   The Computer's "View of the World," 71
Worksheet 30   The Spatial Frequency Domain, 75

Part Four   **Artifacts**

Worksheet 31   Magnetic and RF Field Distortion Artifacts, 77
Worksheet 32   Reconstruction Artifacts, 79

SECTION II
DATA ACQUISITION AND PROCESSING

Part One   **Pulse Sequences**

Worksheet 33   RF Pulse Sequences, 83
Worksheet 34   FID/SE/GE, 85

Part Two   **Data Manipulation**

Worksheet 35   The Fourier Transform, 87
Worksheet 36   Spatial Frequency, 93

Part Three   **Special Procedures**

Worksheet 37   Spin Echo Techniques, 97
Worksheet 38   Gradient Echo Techniques, 101

Part Four   **Sequence Parameters and Options**

Worksheet 39   Purpose of Pulse Sequences, 103
Worksheet 40   Function of Gradient Coils. 105
Worksheet 41   Pulse Sequence Diagrams, 109
Worksheet 42   What is an Image?, 113
Worksheet 43   Image Evaluation Criteria, 115
Worksheet 44   MRI Character, 117

SECTION III
IMAGING PROCEDURES

Worksheet 45   Head, Sagittal Plane, 125
Worksheet 46   Head, Transverse Plane, 127
Worksheet 47   Head, Coronal Plane, 129
Worksheet 48   Vascular Neck, 131
Worksheet 49   Vascular Head, 133
Worksheet 50   C-spine Sagittal Plane, 135
Worksheet 51   C-spine, Transverse and Coronal Planes, 137
Worksheet 52   T-spine, 139
Worksheet 53   L-spine, Sagittal Plane, 143
Worksheet 54   L-spine Transverse Plane, 145
Worksheet 55   Chest, Transverse Plane, 147
Worksheet 56   Chest, Coronal Plane, 149
Worksheet 57   Chest, Sagittal Plane, 151
Worksheet 58   Breast, 153
Worksheet 59   Abdomen, 155

Worksheet 60   Pelvis, Female, 157
Worksheet 61   Pelvis, Male, 159
Worksheet 62   TMJ, 161
Worksheet 63   Shoulder, 163
Worksheet 64   Elbow, 165
Worksheet 65   Wrist, 167
Worksheet 66   Hips, 171
Worksheet 67   Knee, 173
Worksheet 68   Ankle/Foot, 175

SECTION IV
PATIENT CARE AND MRI SAFETY

Worksheet 69   Contrast Agents, 179
Worksheet 70   MRI Energy Fields, 183
Worksheet 71   Human Responses to MRI, 187
Worksheet 72   General Safety Considerations, 189
Worksheet 73   Equipment and Hman Resources, 191
Worksheet 74   Scanning Protocols/Maintenance, 193
Worksheet 75   Safety, 197

SECTION V
APPENDICES

Appendix A   Worksheet Answers, 201
Appendix B   Practice Exam A, 225
Appendix C   Practice Exam B, 235
Appendix D   Answers to Practice Exams, 245

SECTION I

Physical Principles of
Image Formation

PART ONE: INTRODUCTION

Worksheet | 1 |

Historical Trail

1. The earliest medical images were made with visible light, which has higher:

    a. energy than ultraviolet
    b. frequency than x-rays
    c. frequency than gamma rays
    d. energy than RF

2. Which of the following images is not made with electromagnetic radiation?

    a. MR
    b. visible
    c. x-ray
    d. ultrasound

3. The energy range for x-ray imaging is approximately:

    a. 0 to 20 keV
    b. 20 to 50 keV
    c. 20 to 100 keV
    d. 20 to 150 keV

4. Roentgen's discovery of x-rays is dated:

    a. 1893
    b. 1895
    c. 1897
    d. 1999

5. How many volts are in 70 kV?

    a. 700
    b. 7000
    c. 70,000
    d. 700,000

6. Rank the following according to their frequency from lowest to highest:
    (1) visible light
    (2) microwaves
    (3) radiofrequency
    (4) infrared

    a._____
    b._____
    c._____
    d._____

7. Where on the electromagnetic (EM) spectrum will one find diagnostic ultrasound?

    a. between x-rays and ultraviolet
    b. between ultraviolet and infrared
    c. between microwaves and radiofrequency
    d. it's not found on the EM spectrum

8. The range of the visible light spectrum is approximately:

    a. 100 to 500 nm
    b. 300 to 500 nm
    c. 300 to 700 nm
    d. 500 to 1000 nm

9. The approximate range for MR imaging is:

    a. 1 to 10 MHz
    b. 10 to 100 MHz
    c. 100 to 1000 MHz
    d. 1000 to 1,000,000 MHz

10. How many nanometers are in a meter?

    a. 10^0
    b. 10^3
    c. 10^6
    d. 10^9

11. How many cycles per second are there in 50 MHz?

    a. 5×10^3
    b. 5×10^5
    c. 5×10^7
    d. 5×10^9

12. Rank the following according to their wavelength from shortest to longest:
    (1) visible light
    (2) microwaves
    (3) radiofrequency
    (4) infrared

    a._____
    b._____
    c._____
    d._____

13. The first Nobel prize in physics was awarded to Wilhelm C. Roentgen in:

    a. 1895   c. 1901
    b. 1898   d. 1905

14. Which of the following types of images is made with transmitted electromagnetic radiation?

    a. infrared   c. MRI
    b. x-rays   d. visual

15. Rank the following according to their quantum energy from lowest to highest:
    (1) visible light
    (2) microwaves
    (3) gamma rays
    (4) radiofrequency

    a._____
    b._____
    c._____
    d._____

16. Match the following most appropriately:
    (1) mm
    (2) keV
    (3) nm
    (4) MHz

    a. x-rays   _____
    b. RF   _____
    c. ultrasound   _____
    d. visible light   _____

17. Match the following spectral ranges:
    (1) 10 to 100 MHz
    (2) 540 to 1640 kHz
    (3) 300 to 700 nm
    (4) 88 to 108 MHz

    a. AM radio   _____
    b. FM radio   _____
    c. MRI   _____
    d. visible light   _____

18. Magnetic resonance imaging developed from:

    a. nuclear moment spectroscopy
    b. nuclear moment resonance
    c. nuclear magnetic resonance
    d. nuclear resonance spectroscopy

19. The scientist credited with the fundamental discoveries leading to MRI is:

    a. Felix Bloch
    b. Raymond Damadian
    c. Paul Lauterbur
    d. Heinrich Hertz

20. Which of the following images is made with reflected electromagnetic radiation?

    a. ultrasound   c. MRI
    b. x-rays   d. visual

21. The principle reason nuclei have a magnetic field is:

    a. their mass   c. they spin
    b. their charge   d. they precess

22. The first human MR image is credited to:

    a. Felix Block
    b. Paul Lauterbur
    c. Raymond Damadian
    d. Heinrich Hertz

23. Which of the following images is made with emitted electromagnetic radiation?

    a. ultrasound   c. MRI
    b. x-rays   d. visual

24. Match the following to a numeral in the figure below

    a. RF   _____
    b. UV   _____
    c. microwaves   _____
    d. gamma rays   _____

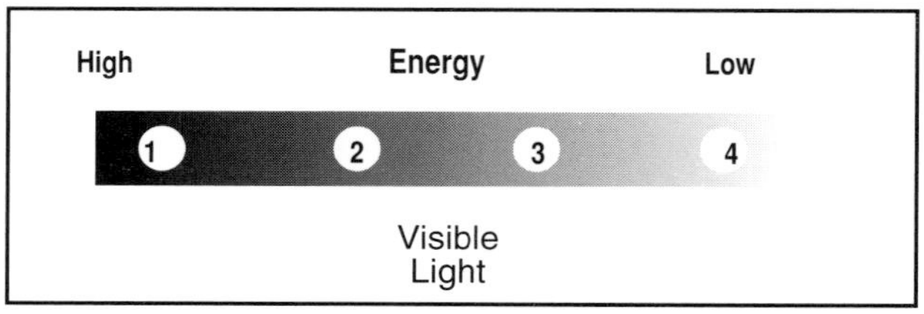

High	Energy	Low
1	2 3	4

Visible
Light

❑ QUESTIONS TO PONDER

25. How many milliseconds (ms) are there in five seconds (s)?

26. Why are the MRI energy fields nonionizing?

27. What does the term orthogonal mean?

28. Where is visible light located on the electromagnetic spectrum relative to x-rays and RF?

Why Do MRI?

1. Which of the following imaging techniques has best spatial resolution?

   a. radioisotope imaging
   b. radiography
   c. computed tomography
   d. magnetic resonance imaging

2. Which of the following would not be considered an advantage of MR imaging?

   a. spatial resolution
   b. contrast resolution
   c. multiplanar imaging
   d. no radiation

3. The contrast resolution available in a radiograph is limited principally by:

   a. linear attenuation coefficient
   b. focal spot size
   c. screen phosphor
   d. collimation

4. Which of the following imaging modalities has best contrast resolution?

   a. radioisotope imaging
   b. radiography
   c. computed tomography
   d. magnetic resonance imaging

5. Which of the following is not one of the four principle RF pulse sequences?

   a. spin echo
   b. spin gradient
   c. gradient recall echo
   d. partial saturation

6. When making a radiograph, the technologist can best influence contrast resolution by:

   a. selecting the small focal spot
   b. selecting the large focal spot
   c. mAs selection
   d. kVp selection

7. Contrast resolution is improved with computed tomography because of:

   a. digital reconstruction
   b. reconstruction by back projection
   c. x-ray beam collimation
   d. x-ray beam filtration

8. Which of the following tissues best represents contrast resolution?

   a. fat-muscle
   b. microcalcifications-glandular
   c. gray matter-white matter
   d. lung-bone

9. ROI in MRI is similar to that in CT. It stands for:

   a. relaxation of interest
   b. relaxation over interpreted
   c. region of interest
   d. region over interpreted

10. Contrast resolution is best described as the ability to:

    a. distinguish among large soft tissues
    b. distinguish among small high density objects
    c. image a large field of view
    d. image a small field of view

11. Contrast resolution in MR imaging is optimized by selection of:

    a. focal spot size   c. mAs
    b. RF pulse sequence   d. kVp

12. Which of the following is not a principle MRI tissue parameter?

    a. linear attenuation coefficient
    b. spin density
    c. longitudinal relaxation
    d. transverse relaxation

13. Spatial resolution is best defined as the ability to:

    a. distinguish among large soft tissues
    b. distinguish among small high density objects
    c. image a large field of view
    d. image a small field of view

14. When making a radiograph, the spatial resolution is principally determined by:

    a. linear attenuation coefficient
    b. focal spot size
    c. screen phosphor
    d. collimation

15. The principle advantage to magnetic resonance imaging is:

    a. spatial resolution
    b. contrast resolution
    c. multiplanar imaging
    d. non-ionizing radiation

16. Which of the following tissue combinations best represents spatial resolution?

    a. fat-muscle
    b. microcalcifications-glandular
    c. gray matter–white matter
    d. lung-bone

17. Multiplanar imaging refers to the ability to:

    a. image orthogonal planes
    b. image orthogonal and oblique planes
    c. image oblique planes
    d. reverse image contrast

18. Which of the following x-ray properties principally determines contrast resolution on a radiograph?

    a. linear attenuation coefficient
    b. spin density
    c. longitudinal relaxation
    d. transverse relaxation

19. When making a radiograph, the radiologic technologist can best influence spatial resolution by:

    a. selecting the small focal spot
    b. selecting the large focal spot
    c. mAs selection
    d. kVp selection

20. The three main components of an MRI imager are:

    a. spin density, longitudinal relaxation, and transverse relaxation
    b. gantry, operating console, and generator
    c. operating console, generator, and coil assembly
    d. gantry, computer, and operating console

21. In MR imaging, the term spin in spin density, refers to spinning:

    a. electrons   c. nuclei
    b. atoms   d. detectors

22. Which of the following atoms is most abundant in the human body?

    a. hydrogen   c. carbon
    b. oxygen   d. nitrogen

23. Which of the following is not included in the gantry of an MRI?

    a. shim coils   c. relaxation coils
    b. gradient coils   d. primary coils

24. The nucleus of a hydrogen atom contains:

    a. one neutron
    b. one proton
    c. one neutron and one proton
    d. two neutrons and two protons

25. Which of the following controls are you likely to find on the console of an MR imager, but not on that of CT?

    a. kVp   c. pulse sequence
    b. mA   d. matrix size

❏ QUESTIONS TO PONDER

26. Compare MRI contrast resolution to radiography and CT.

27. Compare MRI spatial resolution to radiography and CT.

28. Why does calcium appear bright on radiography and dark on MRI?

MRI Briefly

1. Hydrogen makes up approximately _____% of all atoms in the human body?

    a. 20
    b. 40
    c. 80
    d. 90

2. The hydrogen nucleus has a strong magnetic field because it is:

    a. charged
    b. spinning
    c. charged and spinning
    d. charged, spinning and relaxing

3. Prior to placement in a magnet, the net magnetic field of a patient is:

    a. zero
    b. equal to the earth's magnetic field
    c. maximum
    d. equal to B_0

4. Individual nuclear spins are:

    a. B_0
    b. M_0
    c. monopolar
    d. dipolar

5. In vector algebra, which axis is conventionally the vertical axis?

    a. X axis
    b. Y axis
    c. Z axis
    d. it varies

6. A vector quantity is defined as one that has:

    a. spin and charge
    b. mass and charge
    c. magnitude and direction
    d. mass and direction

7. By convention, in MRI the Z axis coincides with:

    a. the vertical axis
    b. either horizontal axis
    c. the axis of the patient
    d. the axis of the static magnetic field

8. In a permanent magnet MR imager the Z axis is:

    a. the long axis of the patient
    b. the lateral axis of the patient
    c. the AP axis of the patient
    d. any of the above

9. The symbol for the primary static magnetic field is:

    a. M_0
    b. B_0
    c. T_0
    d. RF_0

10. The radiation dose associated with a 1.5 T MR imager is:

    a. 0 rads
    b. 1.5 rads
    c. 63 rads
    d. it depends on the RF pulse sequence

11. The MRI signal is weak because:

    a. the static magnetic field is too weak
    b. only one in one million protons are affected
    c. spin precession occurs
    d. there is no ionizing radiation

12. Precession means to:

    a. wobble
    b. rotate
    c. spin
    d. polarize

13. A spinning gyroscope:

    a. becomes polarized
    b. shows net magnetization
    c. induces a magnetic field
    d. has angular momentum

14. Precession occurs when a proton spins:

    a. on the earth
    b. in a magnetic field
    c. on its axis
    d. in an electric field

15. The Larmor equation is stated as:

   a. $\omega = \gamma B$
   b. $\omega = \gamma / B$
   c. $\omega \gamma = B$
   d. $\omega B = \gamma$

16. In the Larmor equation, ω represents the:

   a. frequency of precession
   b. magnetic dipole
   c. gyromagnetic ratio
   d. static magnetic field

17. In the Larmor equation, γ equals the:

   a. frequency of precession
   b. magnetic dipole
   c. gyromagnetic ratio
   d. static magnetic field

18. In the Larmor equation, B equals the:

   a. frequency of precession
   b. magnetic dipole
   c. gyromagnetic ratio
   d. static magnetic field

19. Match the following nuclei to the appropriate gyromagnetic ratio:
   (1) 11.3 MHz/T
   (2) 17.2 MHz/T
   (3) 40.1 MHz/T
   (4) 42.6 MHz/T

   a. hydrogen-1   _____
   b. fluorine-19   _____
   c. phosphorus-31 _____
   d. sodium-23   _____

20. Gyromagnetic ratio is to MRI as:

   a. houndsfield number is to radiography
   b. attenuation coefficient is to diagnostic ultrasound
   c. acoustic impedance is to CT
   d. disintegration constant is to nuclear medicine

21. The units of gyromagnetic ratio are:

   a. MHz (T)
   b. MHz/T
   c. T/MHz
   d. MHz(T2)

22. A 4 T magnet would have a Larmor frequency of approximately:

   a. 20 MHz
   b. 40 MHz
   c. 80 MHz
   d. 160 MHz

23. Hydrogen produces a high MRI signal because of its:

   a. Larmor frequency and gyromagnetic ratio
   b. relative abundance and gyromagnetic ratio
   c. gyromagnetic ratio and spin density
   d. spin density and relaxation time

24. Net magnetization is a:

   a. vector quantity
   b. scaler quantity
   c. spin quantity
   d. relaxation quantity

25. Net magnetization along the B_o axis is represented by:

   a. M_z
   b. B_z
   c. M_o
   d. B_o

26. Net magnetization is:

   a. the total number of proton spins
   b. the density of proton spins
   c. the sum total of polarized spins
   d. resonance between spins

27. Energy transfer from one system to another is most efficient:

   a. during relaxation
   b. during spin precession
   c. at resonance
   d. at equilibrium

28. When a patient is positioned in a static magnetic field for some time, the proton spins are said to be:

   a. relaxing
   b. in phase
   c. saturated
   d. at equilibrium

29. When a proper RF pulse is transmitted into a patient, the proton spins immediately:

   a. spin and precess in phase
   b. precess in phase and flip 180^0
   c. flip 180^0 and equilibrate
   d. equilibrate and spin

30. The primary MR signal is called:

   a. foreign incident detector
   b. free incident detector
   c. free induction detector
   d. free induction decay

31. The FID is a plot of:

    a. signal intensity vs time
    b. signal intensity vs 1/time
    c. spin density vs time
    d. spin density vs 1/time

32. Performing a Fourier transform on an FID results in a plot of:

    a. signal intensity vs time
    b. signal intensity vs 1/time
    c. spin density vs time
    d. spin density vs 1/time

33. To induce means to:

    a. transfer energy
    b. increase signal intensity
    c. cause precession
    d. cause relaxation

34. An NMR spectrum is:

    a. the relaxation of signal intensity
    b. the Fourier transform of an FID
    c. the plot of frequency vs inverse time
    d. induced from the FID

35. Magnetic field gradients are required for:

    a. spectroscopy
    b. MR imaging
    c. spin density assessment
    d. determination of relaxation time

36. Spatial information is obtained during MRI because of:

    a. magnetic field gradients
    b. static magnetic fields
    c. the radiofrequency pulse
    d. spin relaxation

37. Most MR images are formed by:

    a. back projection reconstruction
    b. resonance induction
    c. equilibrium relaxation
    d. two dimensional Fourier transformation

❏ QUESTIONS TO PONDER

38. What is the value of the net magnitization of a patient before being placed in an MR imager?

39. What subsystems move in the gantry of an MR imager?

40. What is M_{xy}?

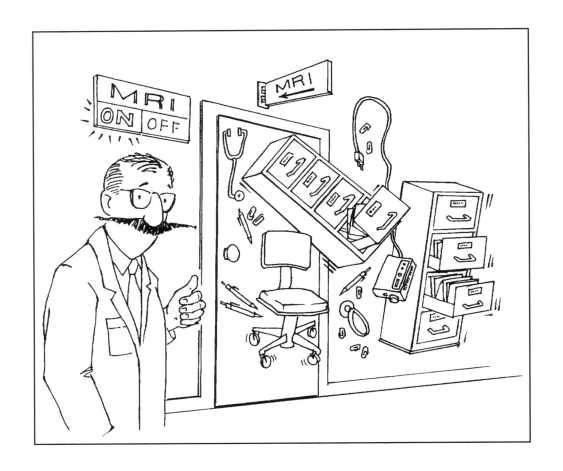

Worksheet 4

Electrostatics

1. The smallest unit of electric charge is contained in:

   a. an electron
   b. a proton
   c. a neutron
   d. an electron or a proton

2. The smallest unit of electric charge is:

   a. that of a neutron
   b. that of an electron
   c. 1/10 the neutron charge
   d. 1/10 the electron charge

3. The American colonial scientist who initiated studies of static electricity is:

   a. Thomas Dalton
   b. Benjamin Franklin
   c. Wilhelm Conrad Roentgen
   d. J. J. Thompson

4. The electron was first identified as a fundamental charged particle by:

   a. Thomas Dalton
   b. Benjamin Franklin
   c. Wilhelm Conrad Roentgen
   d. J. J. Thompson

5. The unit of electric charge is the:

   a. volt
   b. ampere
   c. coulomb
   d. ohm

6. One coulomb is equal to approximately how many electrons?

   a. 1
   b. 10^2
   c. 10^9
   d. 10^{18}

7. The electricity contained in a lightning bolt is measured in:

   a. microcoulombs
   b. millicoulombs
   c. coulombs
   d. kilocoulombs

8. The electric charge associated with electrification by the dry air of winter is measured in:

   a. microcoulombs
   b. millicoulombs
   c. coulombs
   d. kilocoulombs

9. Electrification is defined as:

   a. the induction of electricity
   b. adding or removing electrons
   c. moving electrons in a conductor
   d. propelling electrons in a vacuum

10. Electrification can occur by each of the following, *except*:

    a. induction
    b. contact
    c. friction
    d. precession

11. When one is electrified by walking on a wool carpet, the process is:

    a. precession
    b. contact
    c. friction
    d. induction

12. A bolt of lightning is an example of electrification by:

    a. precession
    b. contact
    c. friction
    d. induction

13. Induction refers to:

    a. a magnetic field generated by rotation
    b. precession in a magnetic field
    c. transfer of energy without touching
    d. interaction of electromagnetic radiation

14. Which of the following would be considered a discrete value, rather than a continuous value?

    a. an electric charge
    b. the electric field
    c. the electromagnetic spectrum
    d. the magnetic field

15. That an electric field exists can be demonstrated by:

   a. precession of a charge in a magnetic field
   b. relaxation of a spin in a magnetic field
   c. a force exerted on a charge
   d. creation of a magnetic field

16. The force of an electric field is:

   a. attractive only
   b. repulsive only
   c. attractive or repulsive
   d. attractive, repulsive, or neutral

17. The intensity of the electric field from an electric charge:

   a. increases as the square of the distance
   b. increases with distance
   c. decreases with distance
   d. decreases as the square of the distance

18. The electric field:

   a. radiates from a positive charge
   b. radiates from a negative charge
   c. is stronger from a positive charge
   d. is stronger from a negative charge

19. The vector nature of the electric field is shown with a:

   a. positive test charge
   b. negative test charge
   c. neutral test charge
   d. positive, negative or neutral test charge

20. The magnitude of an electric field has units of:

   a. newtons
   b. coulombs
   c. newtons per coulomb
   d. coulombs per newton

21. Electric charges are discrete quantities. Electric fields are:

   a. discrete quantities
   b. continuous quantities
   c. interrupted quantities
   d. regulated quantities

22. The four principle laws of electrostatics include:

   a. Tesla's law   c. Coulomb's law
   b. Gauss' law   d. Franklin's law

23. The force created by the electric fields of two electric charges is proportional to the product of the:

   a. two charges and the distance between them
   b. two charges and the inverse of the distance squared between them
   c. distance and the charges
   d. charges and the field strengths

24. In a conductor such as copper, free electrons would be found:

   a. in the middle of the conductor
   b. uniformly distributed throughout the conductor
   c. on the surface of the conductor
   d. in the immediate space surrounding the conductor

25. Free electrons will be found in greatest concentration:

   a. in the space surrounding the conductor
   b. in the middle of the conductor
   c. on the sharpest surface of the conductor
   d. on the most rounded surface of the conductor

26. Electric potential energy is also called:

   a. electric conductance
   b. electric resistance
   c. electromagnetic force
   d. electromotive force

27. The unit of measure of electric potential energy is the:

   a. coulomb   c. volt
   b. ampere   d. ohm

28. The volt is a measure of:

   a. work times charge
   b. work squared times charge
   c. work per unit charge
   d. charge per unit work

❏ QUESTIONS TO PONDER

29. What is static electricity?

30. Illustrate the imaginary lines of the electric field between two electrons.

31. What is electromotive force (emf), and what are its units?

Worksheet | 5 |

Electrodynamics

1. Electrodynamics deals with:

   a. induced electric fields
   b. induced magnetic fields
   c. electricity
   d. electromagnetism

2. Electricity is also called:

   a. electric induction c. electric charge
   b. electomagnetism d. electric current

3. Electricity is important because:

   a. work can be extracted from moving electrons
   b. electric fields are discrete
   c. electric charge is continuous
   d. coulomb force is reduced

4. The unit of electricity is the:

   a. coulomb c. volt
   b. ampere d. ohm

5. One ampere is equal to:

   a. one volt per second
   b. one volt second
   c. one coulomb second
   d. one coulomb per second

6. When applying direct current, as from a battery, electrons flow in:

   a. one direction continuously
   b. one direction intermittently
   c. two directions continuously
   d. two directions intermittently

7. Sixty hertz alternating current will produce 120:

   a. cycles per second
   b. zero crossings per second
   c. positive pulses per second
   d. negative pulses per second

8. When using three-phase electricity:

   a. electrons flow in one direction
   c. the frequency is 180 hertz
   b. electrons flow in both directions
   d. there are 120 zero crossings

9. Which of the following is not a measure of electric impedance?

   a. capacitance c. alternance
   b. inductance d. resistance

10. Impedance which turns electric energy into heat is called:

    a. capacitance c. alternance
    b. inductance d. resistance

11. Resistance in an electric circuit is determined by volts:

    a. times amperes
    b. times coulombs
    c. divided by amperes
    d. divided by coulombs

12. Arrange the following terms in order of increasing resistance (lowest = 1).

    a. conductors   _____
    b. insulators   _____
    c. semiconductors _____
    d. superconductors _____

13. Match the following:
    (1) glass
    (2) niobium
    (3) copper
    (4) silicon

    a. conductors   _____
    b. insulators   _____
    c. semiconductors _____
    d. superconductors _____

14. What material can either allow electrons to flow or resist electron flow?

    a. semiconductor   c. superconductor
    b. conductor   d. insulator

15. Power is defined as:

    a. energy per unit mass
    b. energy per unit charge
    c. the rate of energy use
    d. the rate of coulomb flow

16. Power has units of:

    a. volts per second   c. volts per coulomb
    b. joules per second   d. joules per coulomb

17. Ohm's law is usually stated:

    a. $V = I/R$ c. $V = I^2/R$
    b. $V = IR$ d. $V = I^2R$

18. Electric power is measured in:

    a. coulomb squared   c. ohms
    b. volts squared   d. watts

19. Match the descriptors to a numeral in the following figure.

    a. capacitor   _____
    b. resistor   _____
    c. switch   _____
    d. inductor   _____

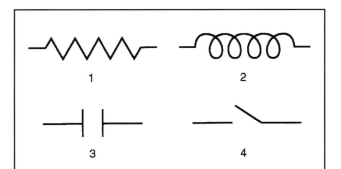

❏ **QUESTIONS TO PONDER**

20. What is electricity?

21. What basic law is primarily used to relate the properties of electricity?

22. What is the difference between a conductor and an insulator?

23. What is a watt?

Magnetism

1. The smallest region of magnetism is called:

   a. magnetic induction
   b. magnetic field
   c. magnetic material
   d. magnetic domain

2. A magnet exists when:

   a. there is an excess of magnetic domains
   b. there is a shortage of magnetic domains
   c. magnetic domains are randomly oriented
   d. magnetic domains are aligned

3. Magnetism, even at the smallest level, is associated with a moving:

   a. voltage   c. mass
   b. resistance   d. charge

4. Atoms that exhibit the strongest magnetism are those with:

   a. paired electrons in outer shells
   b. paired electrons in inner shells
   c. unpaired electrons in half-filled shells
   d. filled electrons shells

5. Which of the following is **not** one of the principle degrees of magnetism?

   a. ferromagnetism   c. paramagnetism
   b. supermagnetism   d. dimagnetism

6. The degree of magnetism of a material is expressed as:

   a. magnetic induction
   b. magnetic flux
   c. magnetic permeability
   d. magnetic susceptibility

7. Common contrast agents used in magnetic resonance imaging are _____ material.

   a. ferromagnetic   c. paramagnetic
   b. supermagnetic   d. dimagnetic

8. The basic law of magnetism states that:

   a. only north poles can exist alone
   b. only south poles can exist alone
   c. both north and south poles can exist alone
   d. neither north or south poles can exist alone

9. If a permanent bar magnet is broken into ever smaller pieces, the result will be:

   a. magnetic induction
   b. electromagnetic induction
   c. monopole
   d. a magnetic domain

10. By convention, the imaginary lines of a magnetic field:

    a. leave the north pole of the magnet
    b. leave the south pole of the magnet
    c. can leave either the north or the south pole
    d. do not have direction

11. One tesla is equal to:

    a. 10 gauss   c. 1000 gauss
    b. 100 gauss   d. 10,000 gauss

12. If a compass is taken to the north pole, its needle will point:

    a. skyward   c. toward the equator
    b. into the earth   d. with a spin

13. The earth has a magnetic field because it:

    a. has mass
    b. revolves about the sun
    c. precesses
    d. rotates

14. Some nonmagnetic materials can be rendered magnetic by:

    a. contact   c. alteration
    b. friction   d. induction

15. The imaginary lines of a magnetic field are called lines of:

    a. intensity   c. precession
    b. induction   d. alignment

16. Which of the following is not a type of magnet used for MRI?

    a. permanent magnet
    b. temporary magnet
    c. resistive magnet
    d. superconducting magnet

17. The scientist associated with establishing electro-magnetic theory is:

    a. Wilhelm C. Roentgen
    b. Karl Gauss
    c. James Clerk Maxwell
    d. Charles Coulomb

18. Of the three fundamental forces:

    a. gravity is the strongest
    b. the electric force is the strongest
    c. the magnetic force is the strongest
    d. electric and magnetic forces are equal

19. Match the following:
    (1) Coulomb's law (2) Gauss' law (3) Ohm's law
    (4) Newton's law

    a. gravitational field _____
    b. electrical resistance _____
    c. electric field   _____
    d. magnetic field   _____

20. Which of the following laws obey the inverse square law?

    a. Newton's law   b. Coulomb's law
    c. Gauss' law   d. all of the above

21. The force exerted by a magnetic field is measured in:

    a. coulombs   b. amperes
    c. newtons   d. tesla

22. A magnetic field is defined as:

    a. the product of a force on a pole
    b. a pole divided by a force
    c. a force divided by a pole
    d. a force divided by a pole squared

23. Magnetic field intensity is measured in:

    a. coulombs   c. amperes per meter
    b. newtons   d. tesla

24. One tesla is equal to:

    a. one newton per ampere-meter
    b. one newton-meter per ampere
    c. one newton-ampere per meter
    d. one newton times ampere-meter

25. A basic law of magnetism states that:

    a. like poles repel, unlike poles repel
    b. like poles repel, unlike poles attract
    c. like poles attract, unlike poles attract
    d. like poles attract, unlike poles repel

❒ QUESTIONS TO PONDER

26. How does the earth's magnetic field strength vary with location?

27. Describe how the north and south poles of a magnet are related as one continuous field.

28. What is the relevance of unpaired electrons to magnetism?

29. The normal isomagnetic exclusion line is 5 gauss. Express this in millitesla.

30. How can one visualize the invisible lines of the magnetic field?

Worksheet | **7** |

Electromagnetism

1. An electron in motion has:

   a. only an electric field
   b. only a magnetic field
   c. both an electric and a magnetic field
   d. neither an electric nor a magnetic field

2. The scientist credited with the foundation of electromagnetism is:

   a. Charles Coulomb c. Hans Oersted
   b. Karl Gauss   d. Nicola Tesla

3. Orstead's experiment showed that _____ in a moving charged particle.

   a. mass increases
   b. the electric field increases
   c. the electric field disappears
   d. a magnetic field appears

4. The magnetic field created by a moving electron is oriented _____ to the electron motion.

   a. opposite   c. perpendicular
   b. parallel   d. oblique

5. An electron moving in a magnetic field experiences a force:

   a. parallel to its motion in the magnetic field
   b. parallel to its motion and against the magnetic field
   c. at right angles to its motion and against the magnetic field
   d. at right angles to both its motion and the magnetic field

6. Using the left hand rule, if the middle finger represents electron motion, the forefinger represents:

   a. the electric field
   b. the gravitational field
   c. the magnetic field
   d. velocity

7. The force exerted on a moving electron by an external magnetic field is given by:

   a. Q/VB   c. QVB
   b. QV/B   d. B/QV

8. The total force on a moving electron due to external electric and magnetic fields is called the _____ force.

   a. Newtonian
   b. Gaussian
   c. Lorentzian
   d. precessional

9. The most intense magnetic field of an electromagnet is:

   a. around the current carrying wire
   b. just off the ends
   c. lateral to the coil
   d. on the axis of the coil

10. A solenoid is a device that:

    a. has an iron core
    b. has a primary and secondary winding
    c. is a helical coil of wire
    d. is a single loop of wire

11. Which of the following devices converts electric energy into mechanical energy?

    a. a generator   c. a transformer
    b. a motor   d. an antennae

12. Which of the following devices converts mechanical energy into electric energy?

    a. a generator   c. a transformer
    b. a motor   d. an antennae

13. The scientist associated with the demonstration of electromagnetic induction is:

   a. Charles Coulomb   c. Nicola Tesla
   b. Hans Oersted   d. Michael Faraday

14. If a magnetic field is moved through a closed loop of wire:

   a. the magnetic field will be intensified
   b. the magnetic field will be reduced
   c. an electric current will be induced
   d. electric resistance will be increased

15. Lenz' law deals with:

   a. the gravitation of force
   b. electromagnetic induction
   c. magnetic attraction
   d. an electric switch

16. The transformer operates on the principle of:

   a. electric field stability
   b. magnetic field stability
   c. electromagnetic precession
   d. electromagnetic induction

17. The radio antennae operates on the principle of:

   a. electric field stability
   b. magnetic field stability
   c. electromagnetic precession
   d. electromagnetic induction

18. The transformer can be operated:

   a. only on direct current
   b. only on alternating current
   c. on direct or alterating current
   d. on neither direct nor alterating current

19. A radio antennae can sense:

   a. a constant magnetic field
   b. only a moving magnetic field
   c. both a constant and a moving magnetic field
   d. neither a constant nor a moving magnetic field

20. Match the circuit elements with the numerals in in the following figure.

   a. transformer _____
   b. battery   _____
   c. diode   _____
   d. inductor   _____

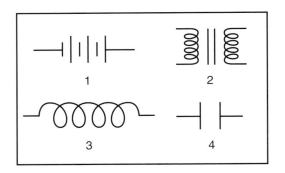

❏ QUESTIONS TO PONDER

21. What is the relationship between a helix, a spiral, and a solenoid?

22. What are eddy currents?

Electromagnetic Radiation

1. A stationary electric charge is associated with a/
   an:

   a. electric field
   b. magnetic field
   c. electromagnetic field
   d. electric current

2. The scientist credited with first describing electromagnetic radiation is:

   a. Wilhelm Conrad Roentgen
   b. Felix Bloch
   c. James Clerk Maxwell
   d. Nikola Tesla

3. Electromagnetic radiation has the properties of a/
   an _____ wave.

   a. amplitude   c. transverse
   b. intensity   d. longitudinal

4. The unit of velocity is the:

   a. hertz   c. meter per second
   b. meter   d. hertz-meter

5. The unit for expressing Planck's constant is the:

   a. joule   c. hertz-second
   b. hertz   d. joule-second

6. Visible light is usually identified by:

   a. energy   c. wavelength
   b. frequency   d. mass

7. The first demonstration of radioemission is credited to:

   a. Wilhelm Conrad Roentgen
   b. Max Planck
   c. Heinrich Hertz
   d. Felix Bloch

8. One meter contains a total of:

   a. 10 nanometers   c. 10^6 nanometers
   b. 10^3 nanometers   d. 10^9 nanometers

9. An MR image is produced from _____ electromagnetic radiation.

   a. reflected   c. emitted
   b. transmitted   d. absorbed

10. When electric charges move in a conductor, a/an
    _____ will be induced.

    a. electric field
    b. magnetic field
    c. electromagnetic field
    d. electric resistance

11. The velocity of electromagnetic radiation, c, is:

    a. 3×10^6 cm per second
    b. 3×10^6 meters per second
    c. 3×10^8 cm per second
    d. 3×10^8 meters per second

12. The classical wave equation has the form of:

    a. velocity = wavelength ÷ frequency
    b. velocity = frequency ÷ wavelength
    c. velocity = wavelength x frequency
    d. velocity x wavelength = frequency

13. Quantum mechanics, first developed by _____,
    describes the action of nuclei and nuclear par-
    ticles.

    a. Albert Einstein
    b. Wilhelm Conrad Roentgen
    c. Felix Bloch
    d. Max Planck

14. In general, electromagnetic radiation of very high energy:

    a. interacts as a photon
    b. interacts as a wave
    c. is absorbed
    d. is reflected

15. RF is usually characterized by:

    a. energy   c. wavelength
    b. frequency   d. mass

16. The visible light imaging window extends from approximately:

    a. 100 to 400 nanometers
    b. 400 to 700 nanometers
    c. 700 to 1000 nanometers
    d. 1000 to 2000 nanometers

17. A visible light image is produced from _____ electromagnetic radiation.

    a. reflected   c. emitted
    b. transmitted   d. absorbed

18. The x-ray imaging window includes photons ranging from:

    a. 10 to 50 eV   c. 30 to 150 eV
    b. 10 to 50 keV   d. 30 to 150 keV

19. The MR imaging window extends from approximately:

    a. 10 to 100 hertz
    b. 10 to 100 megahertz
    c. 100 to 1,000 hertz
    d. 100 to 1,000 megahertz

20. In order to induce an electric current in a secondary coil of wire, the primary coil must be:

    a. supplied with alternating current
    b. supplied with direct current
    c. moved along its axis
    d. moved perpendicular to its axis

21. A photon of electromagnetic radiation consists of electric and magnetic fields oscillating:

    a. in the same plane
    b. 90^0 to one another
    c. constructively placed
    d. destructively placed

22. The unit of wavelength is the:

    a. hertz   c. meter per second
    b. meter   d. hertz-meter

23. In Einstein's famous relativistic equation $E = mc^2$, the energy E is expressed in:

    a. kilogram   c. ergs
    b. electron volts   d. joules

24. Arrange the following electromagnetic radiations according to energy (highest energy = 1).

    a. visible light   _____
    b. radiofrequency   _____
    c. infrared   _____
    d. x-rays   _____

25. X-rays are usually characterized by:

    a. energy   c. wavelength
    b. frequency   d. mass

26. One nanometer is equal to:

    a. 10^3 meter   c. 10^{-6} meter
    b. 10^{-3} meter   d. 10^{-9} meter

27. An x-ray image is produced from _____ electromagnetic radiation.

    a. reflected   c. emitted
    b. transmitted   d. absorbed

28. An x-ray image is possible because of:

    a. wavelike interactions between photons and tissue
    b. particle-like interactions between photons and tissue
    c. reflection of photons and tissue atoms
    d. resonant interactions between photons and tissue atoms

29. An MR imaging room must be shielded to:

    a. keep electromagnetic radiation in the room
    b. keep electromagnetic radiation out of the room
    c. reduce acoustic interference
    d. reduce ionizing radiation levels

30. Electromagnetic radiation is emitted by _____ electric charges.

    a. resting   c. decelerated
    b. moving   d. compound

31. The electric and magnetic fields of electromagnetic radiation oscillate _____ to the direction of velocity:

    a. 0^0 c. 90^0
    b. 45^0 d. 180^0

32. The unit of frequency is the:

    a. hertz   c. meter per second
    b. meter   d. hertz-meter

33. The fundamental equation of quantum mechanics states that:

    a. $h = E\nu$ c. $\nu = Eh$
    b. $E = h\nu$ d. $Eh\nu = 1$

34. On the spectrum of electromagnetic radiation, ultrasound:

    a. has higher energy than visible light
    b. has energy between visible light and radiofrequency
    c. has energy lower than radiofrequency
    d. will not be found

35. Shown below is the model of a photon in which velocity is represented by _____.

    a. A   c. C
    b. B   d. E

36. Wavelength, in the figure below, is represented by _____.

    a. A   c. C
    b. B   d. E

❏ QUESTIONS TO PONDER

37. What does the left superscript and left subscript of calcium $^{40}_{20}\text{Ca}$ mean?

38. What is a covalent bond?

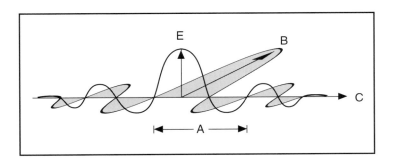

The Gantry/Operating Console

1. The three major components of an MR imager are the:

   a. primary coils, secondary coils, and computer
   b. primary coils, operating console, and computer
   c. gantry, operating console, and computer
   d. gantry, secondary coils, and computer

2. A cryogenic state is one in which:

   a. all motion ceases
   b. all electricity ceases
   c. matter is at magnetic equilibrium
   d. matter is extremely cold

3. The patient couch must be able to accommodate a patient weighing at least:

   a. 70 kg   c. 110 kg
   b. 90 kg   d. 130 kg

4. Relative to the patient the:

   a. RF probe is closer than the shim coils
   b. shim coils are closer than the gradient coils
   c. primary coils are closer than the gradient coils
   d. primary coils are closer than the shim coils

5. In a resistive magnet imager the position of the coils relative to the patient are:

   a. gradient coils, shim coils, primary coils
   b. gradient coils, shim coils, RF probe
   c. shim coils, primary coils, RF probe
   d. primary coils, RF probe, gradient coils

6. When one considers the three principle types of MR imagers, the biggest difference exists in the:

   a. operating console   c. imaging coils
   b. gantry   d. computer

7. There are three sub-assemblies to magnetic resonance imagers:

   a. the primary magnet assembly, cryostat, and secondary magnets
   b. the primary magnet assembly, cryostat, and patient couch
   c. the secondary magnets, patient couch, and cryogenic liquids
   d. the patient couch, primary magnet assembly, and secondary magnets

8. Patient positioning is normally accommodated with:

   a. metric rules
   b. a helical device
   c. two or three gear drives
   d. two or three laser lights

9. From the patient, the order of coil placement is:

   a. RF probe, gradient coil, and shim coil
   b. shim coil, gradient coil, and primary coil
   c. RF probe, primary coil, and shim coil
   d. shim coil, gradient coil, and primary coil

10. A permanent magnet MR imager is:

    a. is constructed of a single large iron magnet
    b. requires two magnet assemblies positioned across the patient aperture
    c. uses permanent magnets for magnetic field gradients
    d. uses permanent magnets to shim the primary magnetic field

11. In the gantry of an MR imager there:

    a. are no moving parts
    b. is a slip ring rotor
    c. are subsystems that move during imaging
    d. are moving electromagnetic coils

12. For superconducting MR imagers:

    a. both the primary magnets and the secondary magnets are at room temperature

    b. both the primary magnets and the secondary magnets are at cryogenic temperature

    c. the primary magnet is at room temperature and the secondary magnets at cryogenic temperatures

    d. the primary magnet is at cryogenic temperature and the secondary magnets at room temperature

13. A cryostat is:
(1) designed to house liquid gases
(2) consists of many concentric chambers
(3) sometimes called a dewar
(4) necessary for all electromagnetic imagers

    a. 1, 2, and 3   c. 2 and 4
    b. 1 and 3   d. all are correct

14. The distinctive features of a permanent magnet gantry are:
(1) an iron yoke
(2) water cooling
(3) brick-like magnets
(4) permanent magnet gradient fields

    a. 1, 2, and 3   c. 2 and 4
    b. 1 and 3   d. all are correct

15. The gantry of an MR imager is rather large principally because of:

    a. the requirement to contain cryogenic gases
    b. the movement of subsystems
    c. the primary and secondary coil systems
    d. the need to accommodate all size patients

16. The patient couch of an MR imager:

    a. need only move in the vertical direction
    b. is moved prior to examination only
    c. is moved during examination only
    d. is moved prior to and during examination

17. Secondary coils include the:

    a. cryostat, primary magnet, and RF probe
    b. primary magnet, RF probe, and shim coils
    c. RF probe, shim coils, and gradient coils
    d. primary magnet, shim coils, and gradient coils

18. Superconducting shim coils:
(1) are usually at room temperature
(2) are positioned in the cryostat
(3) are nearest the patient
(4) are incorporated in actively shielded magnets

    a. 1, 2, and 3   c. 2 and 4
    b. 1 and 3   d. all are correct

19. The electrical current in the primary coils of a resistive electromagnet MR imager is approximately:

    a. 25 mA   c. 2.5 A
    b. 250 mA   d. 25 A

20. A feature of MRI electromagnets that is absent in the permanent magnet system is the:
(1) cooling system
(2) gradient coils
(3) shim coils
(4) gantry

    a. 1, 2, and 3   c. 2 and 4
    b. 1 and 3   d. 4 is correct

21. Normally the:

    a. main coils are inside the gradient coils
    b. main coils are inside the shim coils
    c. shim coils are inside the RF probe
    d. gradient coils are inside the shim coils

22. A resistive electromagnet MR imager will have the following distinct features:
(1) operates at room temperature
(2) requires cooling
(3) consists of multiple separate primary coils
(4) will contain actively shielded shim coils

    a. 1, 2, and 3   c. 2 and 4
    b. 1 and 3   d. all are correct

23. A permanent magnet MR imager is shimmed with:

    a. actively shielded shim coils
    b. cryogenic shim coils
    c. an iron yoke
    d. mechanical adjustment

24. The precision for positioning the patient couch should be within:

    a. ± 1 mm   c. ± 5 mm
    b. ± 3 mm   d. ± 10 mm

25. The operating console of an MR imager appears more like that of:

    a. a radiography unit
    b. computed tomography
    c. a nuclear medicine camera
    d. diagnostic ultrasound

26. Which of the following controls are part of the image acquisition subsystem?
    (1) inversion time
    (2) zoom
    (3) number of views
    (4) collage

    a. 1, 2, and 3   c. 2 and 4
    b. 1 and 3   d. 4

27. Which of the following controls are part of the image processing subsystem?
    (1) pulse sequence
    (2) zoom
    (3) number of views
    (4) profile histogram

    a. 1, 2, and 3   c. 2 and 4
    b. 1 and 3   d. all are correct

28. The operating console of an MR imager contains two general sets of controls:

    a. image acquisition and image processing
    b. magnetic field control and image processing
    c. magnetic field control and image acquisition
    d. patient positioning and image acquisition

29. Which of the following controls are part of the image acquisition subsystem?
    (1) pulse sequence
    (2) repetition time
    (3) slice thickness
    (4) collage

    a. 1, 2, and 3   c. 2 and 4
    b. 1 and 3   d. all are correct

30. Which of the following controls are part of the image processing subsystem?
    (1) highlight
    (2) collage
    (3) cursor on/off
    (4) field of view

    a. 1, 2, and 3   c. 2 and 4
    b. 1 and 3   d. 4

31. Which of the following operating console controls would be part of the start-up subsystem?

    a. CRT control   c. field of view
    b. pulse sequence   d. image annotation

32. Which of the following controls are part of the image acquisition subsystem?
    (1) cursor on/off
    (2) region of interest
    (3) collage
    (4) number of acquisitions

    a. 1, 2, and 3   c. 2 and 4
    b. 1 and 3   d. 4

33. Which of the following controls are part of the image processing subsystem?
    (1) slice thickness
    (2) highlight
    (3) field of view
    (4) collage

    a. 1, 2, and 3   c. 2 and 4
    b. 1 and 3   d. all are correct

34. Computers employed for MRI usually fall into the category of:

    a. personal computers
    b. minicomputers
    c. microcomputers
    d. main frame computers

35. A mathematical computation using floating point numbers is termed a:

    a. bit   c. chomp
    b. byte   d. flop

36. When an MRI computer system is identified as multi-user:

    a. it allows simultaneous multi-patient examination
    b. it allows simultaneous access to the operating console and a viewing console
    c. provides for multiple pulse sequences
    d. is a shared computer concept

37. The two principle characteristics for an MRI computer are:

    a. large size and moveable
    b. large capacity and moveable
    c. large capacity and fast
    d. large range and fast

38. An array processor is a device that:

    a. manipulates flops rather than bits
    b. is hardwired for faster computation
    c. is a special computer program
    d. is the printer used for MRI data

39. Multitasking in an MRI computer refers to:

    a. computing with bits, bytes, or flops
    b. the use of an operating console and physicians console
    c. being able to scan multiple patients at once
    d. allowing computer hardware to be shared by several programs

40. The memory of an MRI computer is measured in:

    a. thousands of bytes
    b. thousands of kilobytes
    c. thousands of megabytes
    d. thousands of gigabits

41. The computer program that controls the operation of the MRI computer is called:

    a. an array processor
    b. a flop
    c. multitasking
    d. an operating system

42. Referring to the figure below, shim coils will be found in:

    a. A   c. C
    b. B   d. D

43. Referring to the figure below, lasers will be found in:

    a. A and B   c. C and D
    b. B and C   d. D and A

44. Referring to the figure below, window/level/zoom controls will be found in:

    a. A   c. C
    b. B   d. D

45. Referring to the figure below, the A/D converter will be found in:

    a. A   c. C
    b. B   d. D

◻ QUESTIONS TO PONDER

46. Why are cryogenic gases required for superconducting MR imagers?

47. What does it mean to reverse the polarity of a magnetic field gradient?

48. What part of the MR. imager reconstructs the image?

49. Why do all MR. imagers have inherent magnetic field inhomogeneities?

50. Where in the gantry are the RF coils positioned?

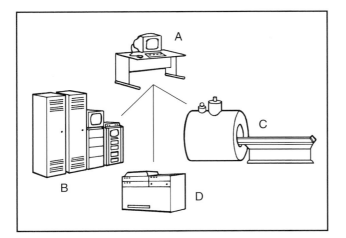

Primary Magnets

1. The maximum field strength obtained with a permanent magnet is approximately:

   a. 0.03 T   c. 0.3 T
   b. 0.15 T   d. 1.5 T

2. The minimum number of individual magnet assemblies required for a permanent magnet MR imager is:

   a. one   c. three
   b. two   d. four

3. The purpose of a pole face is to:

   a. intensify the B_o field
   b. intensify the magnetic field gradients
   c. improve B_o homogeneity
   d. improve magnetic field gradient homogeneity

4. The iron yoke assembly portion of a permanent magnet imager is designed to increase:

   a. the amplitude of the magnetic field gradients
   b. the intensity of B_0
   c. the gyromagnetic ratio
   d. spin density

5. The iron yoke assembly portion of a permanent magnet imager is designed to:

   a. confine the magnetic field gradients
   b. confine the fringe magnetic field
   c. increase the gyromagnetic ratio
   d. increase spin density

6. The iron yoke assembly portion of a permanent magnet imager is designed:

   a. as a frame for the magnetic field gradients
   b. as a frame for mechanical stability
   c. to increase the gyromagnetic ratio
   d. to increase spin density

7. The maximum field intensity obtainable with a resistive electromagnetic imager is approximately:

   a. 0.03 T   c. 0.3 T
   b. 0.15 T   d. 1.5 T

8. One disadvantage to resistive magnet MR imagers is:

   a. electric power consumption
   b. excessive fringe magnetic field
   c. limitation of magnetic field gradients
   d. variation of relaxation times

9. The classic resistive electromagnet for imaging is designed around:

   a. two opposing coils
   b. a concentric iron yoke
   c. a solenoid
   d. four separate coils.

10. Magnetic field homogeneity with resistive electromagnetic imagers ranges from:

    a. 1 to 10 ppm   c. 50 to 100 ppm
    b. 10 to 50 ppm   d. 100 to 500 ppm

11. One advantage to operation of a resistive electromagnet imager is the:

    a. B_0 field can be varied
    b. B_0 field can be turned off
    c. excellent B_0 homogeneity
    d. gyromagnetic ratio can be held constant

12. A principle disadvantage to a resistive electromagnet imager is:

    a. varying relaxation times
    b. B_0 inhomogeneity
    c. ferromagnetic projectiles
    d. electric power consumption

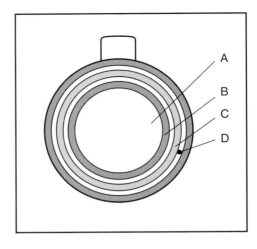

13. Most resistive electromagnetic imagers require power levels of:

    a. 0 to 20 KW   c. 50 to 100 KW
    b. 20 to 50 KW   d. 100 to 200 KW

14. The principle coolant for resistive electromagnet imagers is:

    a. air   c. liquid nitrogen
    b. water   d. liquid helium

15. The principle characteristic of a superconducting electromagnet imager is:

    a. high magnetic field strength
    b. low magnetic fringe field
    c. good patient throughput
    d. poor magnetic field homogeneity

16. An advantage of a superconducting electromagnet imager is:

    a. NMR spectroscopy is possible
    c. constant gyromagnetic ratio
    b. reduced magnetic fringe field
    d. improved patient throughput

17. An advantage of a superconducting electromagnet imager over other types is:

    a. increased signal-to-noise ratio
    b. constant homogeneity coefficient
    c. constant gyromagnetic ratio
    d. low power consumption

18. A disadvantage to a superconducting electromagnet imager is:

    a. intense magnetic fringe field
    b. altered relaxation times
    c. restrictive B_o homogeneity
    d. reduced patient throughput

19. A disadvantage to a superconducting electromagnet imager is:

    a. cryogenic gas is required
    b. reduced signal-to-noise ratio
    c. reduced spatial resolution
    d. changes in relaxation time

20. Which chamber in the figure above contains the superconducting wire?

    a. A   c. C
    b. B   d. D

21. Which chamber in the figure above contains the liquid nitrogen?

    a. A   c. C
    b. B   d. D

22. Which chamber in the figure above contains a vacuum?

    a. A   c. C
    b. B   d. D

23 Which chamber in the figure above contains the RF probe?

    a. A   c. C
    b. B   d. D

❑ **QUESTIONS TO PONDER**

24. How long does it take to turn on the B_o field of an MR imager?

25. Why is a permanent magnet type MRI preferable for developing countries?

26. Identify the types of magnets employed to produce the B_0 field of an MR imager?

27. What is the cause of a quench?

Worksheet

| 11 |

Shim Coils

1. The three classes of secondary MR magnets are:

   a. gradient coils, shim coils, and RF probe
   b. gradient coils, shim coils, and permanent magnet
   c. shim coils, RF coils, and RF probe
   d. head coil, body coil, and surface coil

2. Magnetic field homogeneity is usually expressed as:

   a. parts per million
   b. a range of microtesla
   c. a range of millitesla
   d. a range of tesla

3. A magnetic field homogeneity of ± 20 ppm in a 2 T magnet is equivalent to:

   a. $\pm 2\,\mu T$ c. $\pm 20\,\mu T$
   b. $\pm 4\,\mu T$ d. $\pm 40\,\mu T$

4. A 0.5 T magnet has a field homogeneity of 20 ppm. The Larmor frequency for this imager varies by approximately:

   a. ± 105 Hz   c. ± 420 Hz
   b. ± 210 Hz   d. ± 840 Hz

5. Presently, the best field homogeneity is obtained with:

   a. an actively shielded permanent magnet
   b. a mechanically shimmed resistive electromagnet
   c. a passively shielded superconductive electromagnet
   d. an actively shielded superconductive electromagnet

6. To shim a magnetic field is to make it more:

   a. intense   c. linear
   b. uniform   d. stable

7. The parts per million (ppm) scale:

   a. requires modification according to the type of primary magnet
   b. depends on the type of RF probe employed
   c. depends on the magnetic field strength
   d. is independent of magnetic field strength

8. A 0.5 T magnet has a field homogeneity that varies $\pm 5\,\mu T$. This is equivalent to:

   a. ± 1 ppm   c. ± 10 ppm
   b. ± 2.5 ppm   d. ± 25 ppm

9. A 1 T magnet has 20 ppm field homogeneity. The Larmor frequency for this imager varies by approximately:

   a. ± 105 Hz   c. ± 420 Hz
   b. ± 210 Hz   d. ± 840 Hz

10. Which of the following applications requires the best shimming of the magnet?

    a. conventional spin echo imaging
    b. fast spin echo imaging
    c. echo planar imaging
    d. spectroscopy

11. The magnetic field produced by shim coils is designed to improve the magnetic field produced by:

    a. RF coils   c. RF probe
    b. gradient coils   d. primary coils

12. A homogeneity of ± 1 ppm in a 1 T magnet is a change in magnetic field intensity of:

    a. $\pm 1\,\mu T$ c. ± 1 mT
    b. $\pm 10\,\mu T$ d. ± 10 mT

13. A 1 T magnet has a field homogeneity of $\pm 15\,\mu T$. This is equivalent to:

    a. ± 1.5 ppm   c. ± 15 ppm
    b. ± 10 ppm   d. ± 100 ppm

14. A 1.5 T MR imager has a field homogeneity of 20 ppm. The Larmor frequency for this imager will vary by:

    a. ± 210 Hz   c. ± 630 Hz
    b. ± 420 Hz   d. ± 1260 Hz

15. Shim coils consist of:

    a. a single solenoid type coil with its own power supply
    b. multiple coils each with its own power supply
    c. coils specifically designed for head, body or extremity
    d. coils designed to boost the intensity of the main magnetic field

16. A magnetic field homogeneity of ± 5 ppm in a 1.5T magnet is equal to:

    a. ± 5 µT   c. ± 50 µT
    b. ± 7.5 µT   d. ± 7.5 mT

17. A 1.5 T magnet has a field homogeneity of ± 3 µT. This is equivalent to:

    a. ± 2 ppm   c. ± 20 ppm
    b. ± 3 ppm   d. ± 30 ppm

18. A 2 T MR imager has a field homogeneity of 5 ppm. The Larmor frequency for this imager will vary by:

    a. ± 210 Hz   c. ± 630 Hz
    b. ± 420 Hz   d. ± 840 Hz

19. A magnetic field homogeneity of 10 ppm in a 0.5 T magnet is equivalent to:

    a. ± 1 µT   c. ± 10 µT
    b. ± 5 µT   d. ± 50 µT

20. A 2 T magnet has a field homogeneity of ± 40 µT. This is equivalent to:

    a. ± 1 ppm   c. ± 10 ppm
    b. ± 2 ppm   d. ± 20 ppm

21. When a shim coil is tuned, both the _____ and the _____ of the electric current through the coil is adjusted.

    a. intensity, phase   c. frequency, polarity
    b. phase, frequency   d. polarity, intensity

❑ QUESTIONS TO PONDER

22. What does shim coil adjustment do to image quality?

23. Where are the shim coils, and what is their specific function?

Worksheet 12

Gradient Coils

1. For a superconducting imager the gradient coils are located between the _____ and the _____.

   a. main coils, shim coils
   b. head probe, body probe
   c. body probe, surface coils
   d. body probe, shim coils

2. For a superconducting electromagnet the Z gradient coils are a pair of:

   a. circular coils conducting an AC current
   b. flat coils conducting a DC current of opposite polarity through each
   c. flat coils conducting an AC current
   d. circular coils conducting a DC current of opposite polarity through each

3. Which of the following, shown in the figure below, illustrates the positioning of the X gradient coils in a superconducting MRI?

   a. A   c. C
   b. B   d. D

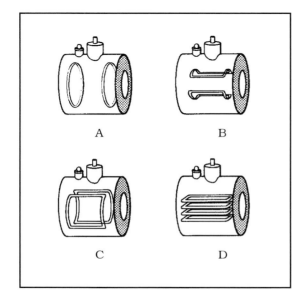

4. Thinner transverse slices can be produced using:
   (1) weaker XY gradient currents
   (2) stronger XY gradient currents
   (3) weaker Z gradient currents
   (4) stronger Z gradient currents

   a. 1, 2, and 3   c. 2 and 4
   b. 1 and 3   d. 4

5. The electronic subsystem that controls the gradient coil is the:

   a. pulse synthesizer   b. pulse programmer
   c. array processor   d. vector synthesizer

6. Magnetic field gradients have intensity up to approximately:

   a. 5 µT/m   c. 5 mT/m
   b. 25 µT/m   d. 25 mT/m

7. If a transverse slice is produced with a superconducting imager the _____ gradient is the slice selection gradient.

   a. X   c. XY
   b. Y   d. Z

8. Which of the following magnetic field gradients is produced by circular gradient coils?

   a. X   c. Z
   b. Y   d. X and Y

9 By convention, in a superconducting MRI the Y axis is:

   a. along the axis of the patient
   b. left to right across the patient
   c. vertically anterior posterior
   d. circular around the patient

10. Shielded gradient coils:
    (1) allow for shorter TR and TE
    (2) reduce eddy currents
    (3) provide higher signal to noise ratio
    (4) improve image contrast

    a. 1, 2, and 3   c. 2 and 4
    b. 1 and 3   d. all are correct

11. Gradient coils are required to carry electric cur-
    rents up to _____ ,with switching times of approxi-
    mately _____ .

    a. 30 mA, 1 μs   c. 30 mA, 1 ms
    b. 30 A, 1 μs   d. 30 A, 1 ms

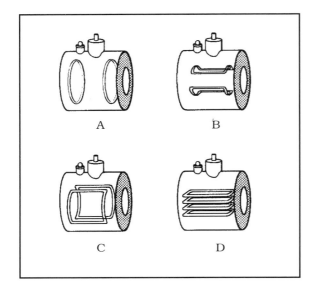

12. Which of the drawings in the above figure prop-
    erly displays Y gradient coils in a superconduct-
    ing MRI?

    a. A   c. C
    b. B   d. D

13. In a superconducting MRI the X axis is:

    a. along the axis of the patient
    b. across the patient from left to right
    c. vertically anterior posteriorly
    d. circular around the patient

14. For transverse images the Y gradient is normally
    the:

    a. slice selection gradient
    b. phase encoding gradient
    c. frequency encoding gradient
    d. shimming gradient

15. The thumping sound which a patient may hear
    during examination is due to the:

    a. primary magnet coils
    b. adjusting shim coils
    c. switching gradient coils
    d. excited RF probe

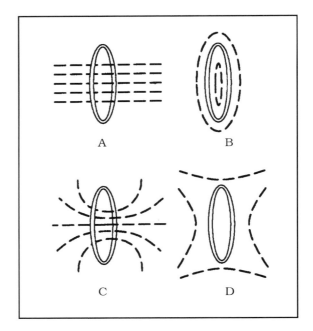

16. Which of the drawings in the figure above best il-
    lustrates the lines of the magnetic field produced
    by a circular coil of wire?

    a. A   c. C
    b. B   d. D

17. The X gradient coils are energized by:

    a. alternating current
    b. direct current of the same polarity
    c. direct current with opposite polarity
    d. alternating current of opposite polarity

18. If the Z gradient is the slice selection gradient, the
    X and Y gradients determine_____ within the slice.

    a. rows and columns
    b. phase and frequency
    c. intensity and polarity
    d. character and location

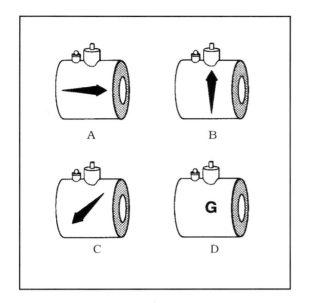

19. Which of the drawings in the figure above best illustrates the Z magnetic field gradient?

   a. A   c. C
   b. B   d. D

20. When the X gradient coils are used for slice selection, the image produced will be:

   a. oblique   c. coronal
   b. transverse   d. sagittal

21. In order to obtain oblique images the three sets of gradient coils must be energized:

   a. sequentially
   c. with varying time delays
   b. segmentally
   d. simultaneously

☐ QUESTIONS TO PONDER

22. What is the relative intensity of the magnetic field gradient compared to the B_0 field?

23. What causes the thump. . . thump. . . thump. . . noise during MRI?

24. How can slice thickness be reduced in the presence of a constant magnetic field gradient?

25. What is rise time?

26. How are oblique views obtained?

Worksheet 13

The RF Probe

1. The RF probe:
   (1) is a primary MRI coil
   (2) operates at high frequency
   (3) shapes the main magnetic field
   (4) can operate as both a transmitter and a receiver

   a. 1, 2, and 3   c. 2 and 4
   b. 1 and 3   d. 4

2. Circular RF probes cannot be employed in super conducting MR imagers because:
   (1) regardless of plane the rotating magnetization would not induce a detectable signal
   (2) the pulse programmer will not accomodate that orientation
   (3) the pulse synthesizer cannot accommodate that orientation
   (4) the B_0 magnetic field is along the axis of the patient

   a. 1, 2 and 3   c. 2 and 4
   b. 1 and   d. 4

3. Homogeneous coils have the distinction of:

   a. transmitting only
   b. receiving only
   c. transmitting and receiving
   d. reducing frequency range

4. In general, the smaller the RF coil the better will be the:
   (1) spatial resolution
   (2) contrast resolution
   (3) signal to noise
   (4) field of view

   a. 1, 2, and 3   c. 2 and 4
   b. 1 and 3   d. all are correct

5. The electronic subsystem that drives the RF probe is called a:

   a. pulse programmer
   b. frequency synthesizer
   c. array processor
   d. ppm divider

6. Quadrature coils are better because they:
   (1) operate over a broader frequency range
   (2) exhibit better signal to noise ratio
   (3) may be polarized
   (4) have better sensitivity

   a. 1, 2, and 3   c. 2 and 4
   b. 1 and 3   d. 4

7. The MR signal emitted by a patient consists of _____ and _____.

   a. linear, circular   c. transmit, receive
   b. gradient, shim   d. signal, noise

8. The principle use of a surface coil is to improve:

   a. field homogeneity
   b. field of view
   c. contrast resolution
   d. spatial resolution

9. Which of the following represents the simplest MRI RF probe?

   a. A   c. C
   b. B   d. D

A   B

C   D

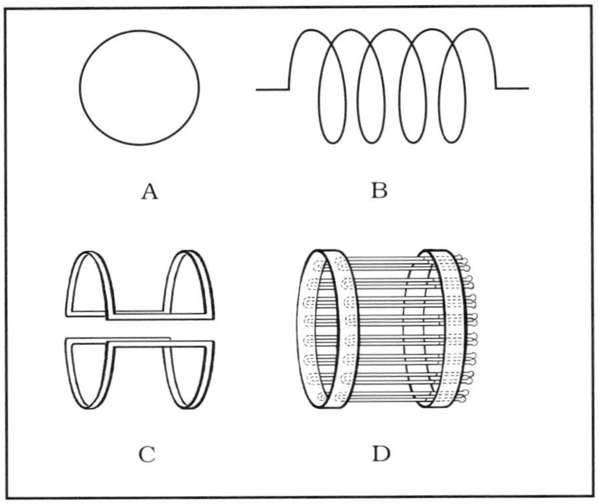

10. An example of a homogeneous coil is:

    a. a spine license plate type coil
    b. a mammography coil
    c. an inner ear coil
    d. a head coil

11. Whereas the detected MR signal comes from _____, MR noise comes from _____.

    a. tissue slice, coil slice
    b. tissue slice, coil volume
    c. tissue volume, coil volume
    d. tissue volume, coil slice

12. Which of the drawings in the above figure represents a birdcage MRI RF probe?

    a. A   c. C
    b. B   d. D

13. Which of the following are always transmit/receive coils?
    (1) the head coil
    (2) a breast coil
    (3) a body coil
    (4) an extremity coil

    a. 1, 2, and 3   c. 2 and 4
    b. 1 and 3   d. all are correct

14. The sensitivity of a circular RF probe is maximum:

    a. inside the circle
    b. outside the circle
    c. adjacent to the wire
    d. perpendicular to the wire

15. Which of the drawings in the figure to the left represents a saddle MRI RF probe?

    a. A   c. C
    b. B   d. D

16. Inhomogeneous coils:

    a. are always linear
    b. are used in conjunction with the body coil
    c. reduce magnetic field homogeneity
    d. are a special kind of gradient coil

17. As a general rule, small MRI coils result in:
    (1) lower signal
    (2) lower noise
    (3) lower contrast
    (4) lower signal to noise ratio

    a. 1, 2, and 3   c. 2 and 4
    b. 1 and 3   d. 4

18. Which of the drawings in the figure to the left represents a solenoid MRI RF probe?

    a. A   c. C
    b. B   d. D

19. A principle disadvantage to using a surface coil is reduced:

    a. field homogeneity   c. contrast resolution
    b. field of view   d. spatial resolution

❒ QUESTIONS TO PONDER

20. In general, when is MRI of bone performed?

21. What should concern the operator performing surface coil imaging?

22. Why are separate transmit and receive coils not routinely used for MRI?

23. What are quadrature coils and where are they used?

24. What is the pixel size when a surface coil field of view (FOV) is 12 cm and the matrix size is 256?

Selecting the Imager

1. Planning for installation of an MRI is more difficult than for radiographic or fluoroscopic equipment because of:

   a. cost
   b. personnel requirements
   c. siting requirements
   d. radiation control

2. Resistive magnet imagers have the following characteristics:
   (1) cost less than one million dollars
   (2) 80 kW power required
   (3) a 2 m magnetic fringe field
   (4) up to 1 tesla field strength

   a. 1, 2, and 3   c. 2 and 4
   b. 1 and 3   d. all are correct

3. Which of the following are advantages to a resistive magnet MR imager?
   (1) low capital cost
   (2) low operating cost
   (3) can be turned off
   (4) no cooling required

   a. 1, 2, and 3   c. 2 and 4
   b. 1 and 3   d. all are correct

4. The 0.5 mT fringe magnetic field does not extend beyond _____ of a permanent magnet imager.

   a. 1 meter   c. 10 meters
   b. 5 meters   d. 20 meters

5. Establishing an MRI facility is a three-stage process which should follow the sequence:

   a. select the imager, identify the site, design the facility
   b. identify the site, design the facility, select the imager
   c. select the imager, design the facility, identify the site
   d. identify the site, select the imager, design the facility

6. Superconducting magnets have the following characteristics:
   (1) 1.5 tesla field strength
   (2) cost over a million dollars
   (3) low power requirements
   (4) large magnetic fringe field

   a. 1, 2, and 3   c. 2 and 4
   b. 1 and 3   d. all are correct

7. MR image quality:

   a. is independent of the means of producing the magnetic field
   b. is proportional to magnetic field strength
   c. improves with increasing Larmor frequency
   d. is improved by more intense magnetic fringe fields

8. A superconducting magnet MR imager has the principle advantage of high:

   a. capital cost   c. B_0 field
   b. cryogen cost   d. power consumption

9. The principle disadvantage of a permanent magnet MR imager is:

   a. weight
   b. fringe magnetic field
   c. cost
   d. limited B_0

10. The application of magnetic resonance spectroscopy:
    (1) should be considered for all new facilities
    (2) should be considered only for research institutions
    (3) is of considerable clinical efficacy
    (4) is lacking in clinical application

    a. 1, 2, and 3   c. 2 and 4
    b. 1 and 3   d. all are correct

11. The principle advantage to a permanent magnet imager is:

    a. intense B_0 field
    b. lightweight and mobile
    c. negligible fringe field
    d. variable field strength

12. A superconducting magnet MR imager has the principle disadvantage of:

    a. high field strength
    b. poor field homogeneity
    c. high power consumption
    d. intense magnetic fringe field

13. Of the magnets available for MR imaging the only one that can be conveniently turned off at night is the:

    a. permanent magnet
    b. resistive electromagnet
    c. Larmor magnet
    d. superconducting electromagnet

14. If magnetic resonance spectroscopy is planned:

    a. a permanent magnet imager must be selected
    b. a resistive magnet imager must be selected
    c. a superconducting magnet imager must be selected
    d. the size of the facility must be increased

15. Which of the following are advantages to permanent magnet imagers?
    (1) low capital cost
    (2) low operating cost
    (3) negligible fringe field
    (4) intense B_0 field

    a. 1, 2, and 3   c. 2 and 4
    b. 1 and 3   d. all are correct

16. A superconducting magnet MR imager has the following characteristics:
    (1) high capital cost
    (2) good field homogeneity
    (3) intense magnetic fringe field
    (4) negligible power consumption

    a. 1, 2, and 3   c. 2 and 4
    b. 1 and 3   d. all are correct

17. The principle reason for using a superconducting electromagnet for MRI is its intense:

    a. B_0 field
    b. transient magnetic field
    c. RF field
    d. fringe magnetic field

18. A permanent magnet imager has the following characteristics:
    (1) field strength up to 0.3 tesla
    (2) cost exceeding one million dollars
    (3) negligible fringe field
    (4) approximately 80 kW power required

    a. 1, 2, and 3   c. 2 and 4
    b. 1 and 3   d. all are correct

19. A resistive magnet imager has the principle advantage of:

    a. low B_0 field   c. low operating cost
    b. low capital cost   d. low fringe field

20. Which magnet in the figure below has a cryostat?

    a. A   c. C
    b. B   d. D

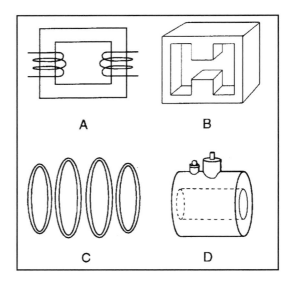

21. Which magnet in the figure above uses the most electricity?

    a. A   c. C
    b. B   d. D

22. Which magnet in the figure above requires no electricity?

    a. A   c. C
    b. B   d. D

❑ QUESTIONS TO PONDER

23. How is the magnetic fringe field determined for an MRI facility?

24. If service were very remote, what type of MR imager would you buy?

Worksheet | 15 |

Locating the MR Imager

1. The location of an MR imager is restricted to:
   (1) new construction
   (2) an existing building
   (3) a temporary building
   (4) a mobile van

   a. 1, 2, and 3   c. 2 and 4
   b. 1 and 3   d. all are correct

2. One advantage to new construction for the siting of an MR imager is that:

   a. shielding of the fringe magnetic field may be unnecessary
   b. stability of the RF system will be improved
   c. cost of RF shielding is reduced
   d. exclusion area is less bothersome

3. Site preparation costs are probably lowest when one chooses:

   a. an existing building
   b. new construction
   c. mobile van
   d. a temporary but fixed location

4. A mobile van is an attractive alternative to locating an imager because of:
   (1) the experience gained by all
   (2) no long term commitment
   (3) cost
   (4) magnetic field strength

   a. 1, 2, and 3   c. 2 and 4
   b. 1 and 3   d. all are correct

5. The fringe magnetic field of an MR imager can influence devices such as:
   (1) x-ray tubes
   (2) cathode ray tubes
   (3) hospital paging systems
   (4) gamma cameras

   a. 1, 2, and 3   c. 2 and 4
   b. 1 and 3   d. all are correct

6. The intensity of a fringe magnetic field:

   a. increases inversely with the intensity of the B_0 field
   b. increases proportionately with the intensity of the B_0 field
   c. is inversely proportional with the transient magnetic field
   d. increases with intensity of the transient magnetic field

7. One advantage of using superconducting shim coils for fringe magnetic field shielding is the:

   a. improvement in B_0 homogeneity
   b. increase in Larmor frequency
   c. more intense transient magnetic fields
   d. less cryogen consumption

8. One shields an MR imager principally to:

   a. make B_0 more homogeneous
   b. improve signal strength
   c. keep electromagnetic radiation out of the room
   d. keep electromagnetic radiation within the room

9. Devices whose operation can be impaired by the fringe magnetic field of an MR imager include those based on:

   a. centripetal force effects
   b. electron vacuum tubes
   c. rotating flywheels
   d. photographic emulsions

10. The intensity of a fringe magnetic field can be reduced by:
    (1) lowering the Larmor frequency
    (2) active shielding
    (3) transient field effects
    (4) passive shielding

    a. 1, 2, and 3   c. 2 and 4
    b. 1 and 3   d. all are correct

39

11. When a large mass of iron is adjacent to the MR examination room, the:
    (1) fringe magnetic field distortion can occur
    (2) fringe magnetic field may be intensified
    (3) B_0 magnetic field may be distorted
    (4) B_0 magnetic field may be intensified

    a. 1, 2, and 3   c. 2 and 4
    b. 1 and 3   d. 4

12. The RF shield designed into the walls of an MR imaging suite are sometimes called a/an:

    a. Larmor barrier
    b. spin density trap
    c. Faraday cage
    d. induced residence

13. The effect of a fringe magnetic field on electron motion in a vacuum is to:

    a. accelerate the electron
    b. decelerate the electron
    c. stop the electron
    d. bend the electron

14. A general rule of thumb holds that the fringe magnetic field will be reduced to half its distance by adding _____ iron in the wall.

    a. 1 mm   c. 1 cm
    b. 5 mm   d. 5 cm

15. A mass of moving iron adjacent to an MR imaging room can cause bothersome distortions in:

    a. B_0 field homogeneity
    b. RF field homogeneity
    c. gradient magnetic field intensity
    d. fringe magnetic field intensity

16. RF shielding of an MRI room can be done with:
    (1) aluminum sheets
    (2) aluminum wire mesh
    (3) copper sheets
    (4) copper wire mesh

    a. 1, 2, and 3   c. 2 and 4
    b. 1 and 3   d. all are correct

17. RF shielding of an MRI room must cover:
    (1) all walls
    (2) the floor
    (3) all doors and windows
    (4) the ceiling

    a. 1, 2, and 3   c. 2 and 4
    b. 1 and 3   d. all are correct

18. Adding iron to the wall of an MR imaging room is an example of:

    a. active shielding
    b. passive shielding
    c. Larmor shielding
    d. spin density shielding

19. According to the Federal Communications Commission the RF band of electromagnetic radiation ranges from:

    a. 30 kHz to 30 GHz
    b. 3 kHz to 30 GHz
    c. 30 kHz to 300 GHz
    d. 3 kHz to 300 GHz

20. Which of the following is least likely to be influenced by a fringe magnetic field?

    a. a credit card
    b. a gamma camera
    c. an electron microscope
    d. a computed tomography imager

21. An MR imager can be actively shielded by:

    a. fastening iron to the magnet
    b. increasing the cryogen capacity
    c. employing shim coils of the same polarity
    d. employing shim coils of opposite polarity

22. RF employed for MRI covers the approximate range of:

    a. 1 to 10 MHz   c. 10 to 1000 MHz
    b. 10 to 100 MHz   d. 1 to 100 MHz

23. Rank the following devices according to their sensitivity to the fringe magnetic field. (1 = most sensitive)

    a. cathode ray tube _____
    b. electron microscope_____
    c. credit cards _____
    d. computers _____

◻ QUESTIONS TO PONDER

24. Why are MRI rooms shielded?

25. Why is the fringe field of a permanent magnet system always less than that of a superconducting system?

Worksheet | 16

Designing the Facility

1. The room for storing cryogens must be:

   a. refrigerated
   b. secured
   c. RF protected
   d. magnetic field protected

2. Once a superconducting imager is at field the power required for the primary magnet coils is approximately:

   a. 0 kW   c. 20-30 kW
   b. 10-20 kW   d. 60-80 kW

3. Construction materials for an MR facility may include:
   (1) standard nails and wood studs
   (2) fiberglass reinforcing bars
   (3) electrical supplies of aluminum or ceramic
   (4) iron reinforcing bar in the concrete slab

   a. 1, 2, and 3   c. 2 and 4
   b. 1 and 3   d. 4

4. Computer facilities must be housed in a controlled environment between:

   a. 15° and 18° C at a relative humidity of not more than 20%
   b. 18° and 20° C at a relative humidity of not more than 40%
   c. 18° and 20° C at a relative humidity of not more than 20%
   d. 15° and 18° C at a relative humidity of not more than 40%

5. Resistive electromagnets are usually:

   a. cooled with water
   b. cooled with liquid nitrogen
   c. cooled with liquid helium
   d. not cooled

6. Metal detection for visitors and patients is:
   (1) unnecessary
   (2) required
   (3) done with x rays
   (4) to protect against projectiles

   a. 1, 2, and 3   c. 2 and 4
   b. 1 and 3   d. 4

7. The power requirements of a resistive type magnetic imager are approximately:

   a. 0 kW   c. 20-30 kW
   b. 10-20 kW   d. 60-80 kW

8. The following building materials are acceptable for an MRI facility:
   (1) aluminum or polyvinylcloride electrical conduit
   (2) brass or copper plumbing fixtures
   (3) incandescent room lamps
   (4) fluorescent room lamps

   a. 1, 2, and 3   c. 2 and 4
   b. 1 and 3   d. 4

9. The following types of electromagnets require special cooling:
   (1) resistive
   (2) permanent
   (3) superconductive
   (4) RF

   a. 1, 2, and 3   c. 2 and 3
   b. 1 and 3   d. 4

10. Superconducting electromagnets are always:

    a. cooled with water
    b. cooled with liquid nitrogen
    c. cooled with liquid helium
    d. not cooled

11. Access to the MR imaging room should be planned to accommodate:
    (1) many outpatients
    (2) mostly outpatients
    (3) patients in distress
    (4) patients asleep

    a. 1, 2, and 3   c. 2 and 4
    b. 1 and 3   d. 4

12. Construction of an MRI site should consider:
    (1) exclusion of large metal objects
    (2) the proximity of x-ray machines
    (3) a vibration free structure
    (4) a ground level facility

    a. 1, 2, and 3   c. 2 and 4
    b. 1 and 3   d. all are correct

13. Constant examination room temperature is especially critical for:

    a. a permanent magnet imager
    b. a resistive electromagnet imager
    c. a superconducting electromagnet imager
    d. surface coil imaging

14. Permanent magnet imagers are usually:

    a. cooled with water
    b. cooled with liquid nitrogen
    c. cooled with liquid helium
    d. not cooled

15. Cryogen off gas from a superconducting electromagnet MRI must be vented to the outside:

    a. in order to maintain a constant temperature in the room
    b. to keep from burning MRI operators
    c. to ensure plenty of oxygen
    d. so it can be recovered

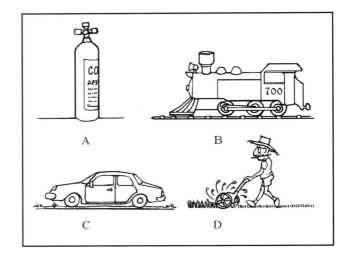

A   B

C   D

16. Which of the above is of most concern when siting an MR imager?

    a. A   c. C
    b. B   d. D

☐ QUESTIONS TO PONDER

17. Why is the computer room temperature and humidity controlled?

18. What is the source of cryogenic helium and nitrogen?

Quantum Mechanical Description

1. A nuclear property described by quantum mechanics is:

   a. mass   c. spin
   b. charge   d. precession

2. An MRI signal is observed when:

   a. nuclear spins are energized
   b. spin density is established
   c. nuclear spins relax
   d. the gyromagnetic ratio is lengthened

3. Which of the following will induce a magnetic field?

   a. a resting electron   c. a spinning neutron
   b. a resting proton   d. a spinning proton

4. Nuclei with even numbers of neutrons and even numbers of protons are likely to have a spin quantum number of:

   a. 0   c. 1
   b. 1/2   d. 3/2

5. When a B_0 field is present, nuclei prefer to:

   a. precess clockwise
   b. precess counter-clockwise
   c. be in a low energy state
   d. be in a high energy state

6. The degree of nuclear spin is identified by:

   a. precessional frequency
   b. magnetic field intensity
   c. spin density
   d. spin quantum number

7. The intensity of a nuclear magnetic moment is determined by:
   (1) mass
   (2) charge
   (3) spin frequency
   (4) spin density

   a. 1, 2, and 3   c. 2 and 4
   b. 1 and 3   d. all are correct

8. The spin quantum number determines:

   a. magnetic field intensity
   b. gyromagnetic ratio
   c. the number of ways a nucleus can spin
   d. the Larmor frequency

9. In MRI, we cause some nuclei to flip from the low energy state to the high energy state by using:

   a. a short T1   c. an RF pulse
   b. a short T2   d. a gyromagnetic ratio

10. Which of the following is not an allowed value for spin quantum number?

    a. 0   c. 1/2
    b. 1/4   d. 1

11. When nuclear spins are at equilibrium with an external magnetic field:

    a. more spins will be in a low energy state
    b. more spins will be in a high energy state
    c. spin density will be lower
    d. spin density will be higher

12. Hydrogen has a spin quantum number of:

    a. 0   c. 1
    b. 1/2   d. 3/2

13. If there is no external magnetic field:

    a. precession is random
    b. rotation is random
    c. each spin state will have the same energy
    d. each spin state will have a different energy

14. How many allowed spin states are there for hydrogen?

    a. 0   c. 2
    b. 1   d. 3

15. In the presence of an external magnetic field:

    a. precession is random
    b. rotation is random
    c. each spin state will have the same energy
    d. each spin state will have a different energy

16. Nuclear spins are at equilibrium when:

    a. they are randomly positioned
    b. they are positioned perpendicular to B_0
    c. more are aligned with B_0
    d. more are aligned against B_0

17. The magnetic field associated with the nucleus of hydrogen is termed:

    a. gyromagnetic field
    b. nuclear magnetic field
    c. gyromagnetic moment
    d. nuclear magnetic moment

18. Quantum mechanics is that branch of physics that describes very:

    a. large objects   c. high energies
    b. small objects   d. low energies

19. In an energized state, more nuclear spins are:

    a. aligned with the external magnetic field
    b. aligned against the external magnetic field
    c. spin faster
    d. spin slower

20. When nuclear spins are at equilibrium with an external magnetic field, more nuclei:

    a. are in a high energy state
    b. are in a low energy state
    c. spin
    d. rotate

21. Every nucleus is known to have:
    (1) mass
    (2) charge
    (3) spin
    (4) frequency

    a. 1, 2, and 3   c. 2 and 4
    b. 1 and 3   d. all are correct

22. The magnetic field associated with a spinning charged particle is given the special name:

    a. magnetic field
    c. nuclear magnetic field
    b. electric field
    d. nuclear magnetic moment

23. Nuclear spin quantum numbers take on _____ values.

    a. continuous   c. integer
    b. half integer   d. exponential

24. Classical mechanics is that branch of physics which describes very:

    a. large objects   c. high energies
    b. small objects   d. low energies

25. Because nuclei spin on an imaginary axis, they:

    a. produce an electric field
    b. induce a magnetic field
    c. become energized
    d. reach equilibrium

26. Classical mechanics is attributed principally to _____, while quantum mechanics is attributed to _____.

    a. Wilhelm Conrad Roentgen, Felix Bloch
    b. Isaac Newton, Max Planck
    c. Albert Einstein, Felix Bloch
    d. James Clerk Maxwell, Heinrich Hertz

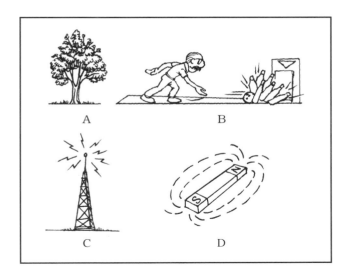

27. Which of the drawings in the above figure most closely relates to quantum mechanics?

    a. A   c. C
    b. B   d. D

28. What is the relevance of atomic number (Z) and atomic mass number (A) in MRI?

29. How can one determine the gyromagnetic ratio of any given element in the body?

30. If one in a million protons participate in MRI, how many are involved in a 1 cc sample?

31. What is meant by coherence and incoherence?

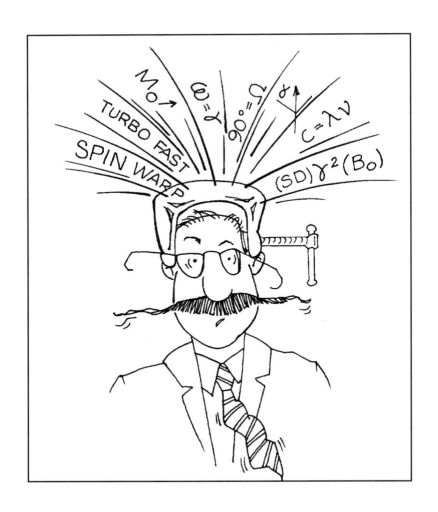

Worksheet $\boxed{18}$

Classical Mechanical Description

1. The symbol for the Greek letter mu is:

   a. γ c. σ
   b. Σ d. μ

2. A gyroscope wobbles because of an interaction between:

   a. mass and charge   c. charge and charge
   b. mass and mass   d. charge and spin

3. The Larmor equation is best stated as:

   a. $\omega\gamma = B$ c. $\omega = \gamma B$
   b. $\omega B = \gamma$ d. $\omega\gamma B = 1$

4. In the Larmor equation, B is the:

   a. gyromagnetic ratio in megahertz
   b. frequency of precession in megahertz
   c. magnetic field intensity in tesla
   d. magnetic field intensity in megahertz per tesla

5. Gyromagnetic ratio in MRI is analogous to the:

   a. wavelength of visible light
   b. mass of an object
   c. disintegration constant in nuclear medicine
   d. energy of a photon

6. In the absence of an external magnetic field the direction of a nuclear magnetic moment will:

   a. be random   c. be straight down
   b. be straight up   d. spin

7. A nuclear magnetic moment in the presence of an external magnetic field interacts by:

   a. mass and mass
   b. charge and charge
   c. magnetic field and magnetic field
   d. magnetic field and electric field

8. In the Larmor equation, omega (ω) is the:

   a. gyromagnetic ratio in megahertz
   b. gyromagnetic ratio in megahertz per tesla
   c. frequency of precession in megahertz
   d. frequency of precession in megahertz per tesla

9. The gyromagnetic ratio for a given nucleus:

   a. is determined by the magnetic field
   b. has a specific value
   c. varies with the frequency of precession
   d. has units of tesla per megahertz

10. A 1.5 tesla MR imager has an operating frequency of:

    a. 11 megahertz   c. 42 megahertz
    b. 21 megahertz   d. 63 megahertz

11. Bar magnets tend to align:

    a. parallel to each other
    b. perpendicular to each other
    c. opposite each other
    d. in a rotating fashion

12. The wobbling motion of a spinning gyroscope is called:

    a. induction   c. translation
    b. precession   d. rotation

13. In the Larmor equation, gamma (γ) is the:

    a. gyromagnetic ratio in megahertz
    b. gyromagnetic ratio in megahertz per tesla
    c. frequency of precession in megahertz
    d. frequency of precession in megahertz per tesla

14. The gyromagnetic ratio for hydrogen has a value of approximately:

    a. 13 megahertz per tesla
    b. 21 megahertz per tesla
    c. 42 megahertz per tesla
    d. 63 megahertz per tesla

15. A 500 megahertz NMR magnet will have a magnetic field strength of:

    a. 1.5 tesla   c. 6.7 tesla
    b. 2.4 tesla   d. 11.7 tesla

16. Which of the drawings in the following figure most closely relates to classical mechanics?

    a. A   c. C
    b. B   d. D

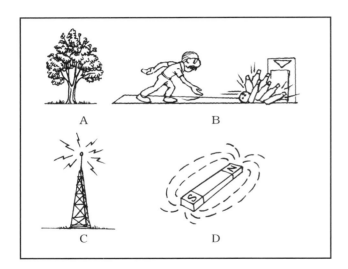

QUESTIONS TO PONDER

17. How long will proton spins align with the B_0 field and precess in the absence of an RF pulse?

18. What position are the proton spins relative to each other in the presence of B_0?

19. When is the maximum intensity of any MRI signal?

20. Why do spins dephase after net magnetization is flipped onto the XY plane?

21. Why does fat (lipid) usually appear bright?

Worksheet 19

Net Magnetization

1. Net magnetization is defined as the:

   a. number of nuclei in a voxel
   b. number of nuclei in a patient
   c. total number of spins
   d. sum of nuclear magnetic moments

2. When M equals zero, this indicates that nuclear magnetic moments:

   a. are arranged parallel
   b. are arranged opposite
   c. are arranged randomly
   d. have disappeared

3. Which of the vector diagrams in the following figure properly represents net magnetization at equilibrium?

   a. A   c. C
   b. B   d. D

4. M_0 is proportional to:

   a. the square of the spin density
   b. gyromagnetic ratio
   c. B_0
   d. T

5. The symbol for net magnetization is:

   a. E_0 c. M
   b. B_0 d. μ

6. Which of the drawings in the following figure represents the proper way to render a three-dimensional coordinate system?

   a. A   c. C
   b. B   d. D

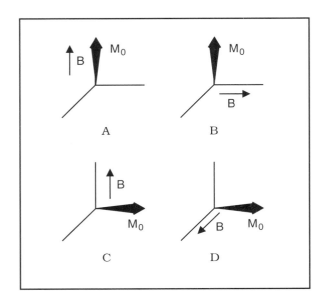

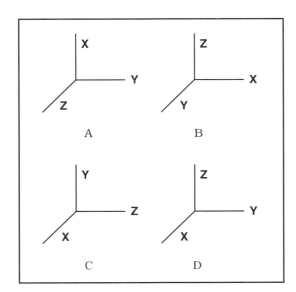

7. Net magnetization at equilibrium, M_0, is important to MRI because its value determines:

    a. T1 relaxation time
    b. T2 relaxation time
    c. precessional frequency
    d. signal intensity

8. M_0 is inversely proportional to:

    a. spin density   c. B
    b. gyromagnetic ratio   d. T

9. Net magnetization is rotated or flipped from the Z axis in order to:

    a. detect it
    b. induce spin density
    c. stimulate relaxation time
    d. measure precessional frequency

10. The symbol for nuclear magnetic moment is:

    a. E   c. M
    b. B   d. μ

11. A vector diagram is a rendering of something that has:

    a. charge and mass
    b. mass and quantity
    c. quantity and direction
    d. direction and spin

12. M_0 is proportional to:

    a. spin density   c. B^2
    b. gyromagnetic ratio   d. T

13. The difference in MR signal intensity from one tissue to another is influenced by:

    a. spin density   c. B
    b. gyromagnetic ratio   d. T

14. MR signal intensity is directly proportional to:
    (1) spin density
    (2) gyromagnetic ratio
    (3) gyromagnetic ratio squared
    (4) spin density squared

    a. 1, 2, and 3   c. 2 and 4
    b. 1 and 3   d. all are correct

15. In the absence of an external magnetic field, net magnetization has a:

    a. maximum value   c. value of zero
    b. minimum value   d. value that varies

16. When tissues are placed in an external magnetic field, individual nuclear magnetic moments:

    a. align instantly   c. become unaligned
    b. align over time   d. are unaffected

17. M_0 is proportional to:

    a. the square of the spin density
    b. the square of the gyromagnetic ratio
    c. B^{-2}
    d. T^{-2}

18. Of all of the net magnetization vectors, the one which cannot be measured is:

    a. M_0 c. M_y
    b. M_x d. M_z

19. Which diagram in the following figure represents net magnetization at equilibrium in a superconducting MR imager?

    a. A   c. C
    b. B   d. D

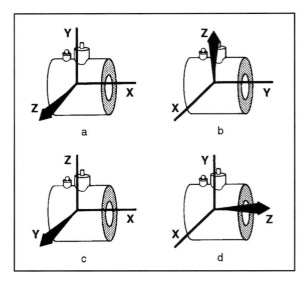

☐ QUESTIONS TO PONDER

20. Why does the Larmor frequency vary throughout the patient during MR imaging?

21. Why can a magnetic field be altered by another magnetic field?

22. What is the value of net magnetization, M_0, when the patient is removed from the magnet?

23. What is meant by spin saturation?

24. What tissue usually generates the most intense MRI signal and therefore the brightest pixels? The least intense and darkest pixels?

Worksheet | 20

Reference Frames

1. In either frame of reference employed in MRI, the Z axis is always the direction of the:

   a. relaxation time
   b. spin density
   c. external magnetic field
   d. gyromagnetic ratio

2. The laboratory frame of reference is sometimes called the _____ frame.

   a. rotating
   b. translating
   c. precessing
   d. stationary

3. In a superconducting magnet, the Z axis is:

   a. vertical
   b. parallel to B_0
   c. perpendicular to B_0
   d. horizontal and perpendicular to B_0

4. In order to flip net magnetization from the Z axis, one must employ:

   a. the proper T1 relaxation time
   b. the proper T2 relaxation time
   c. a static magnetic field of proper frequency
   d. a rotating magnetic field of proper frequency

5. In the rotating frame of reference, an observer:

   a. is in that frame
   b. is outside of that frame
   c. oscillates in and out of that frame
   d. is in the adjacent frame

6. The available permanent magnet imagers have a/an _____ B_0 field.

   a. vertical
   b. longitudinal
   c. transverse
   d. oblique

7. Energy is most efficiently transferred from one system to another at:

   a. precession
   b. resonance
   c. relaxation
   d. spin density

8. Vector diagrams used to illustrate MRI principles are in the _____ frame.

   a. laboratory
   b. stationary
   c. rotating
   d. oblique

9. The maximum MRI signal is produced following:

   a. a 0^0 RF pulse
   b. an alpha RF pulse
   c. a 90^0 RF pulse
   d. a 180^0 RF pulse

10. In the rotating frame, the net magnetization vector:

    a. precesses at the Larmor frequency
    b. does not precess
    c. decays with T1 relaxation
    d. decays with T2 relaxation

11. In MRI, the flip of net magnetization from the Z axis is accomplished by a:

    a. laboratory frame
    b. rotating frame
    c. radiofrequency pulse
    d. magnetic field gradient

12. Which of the drawings in the following figure represents a 135° flip angle?

a. A   c. C
b. B   d. D

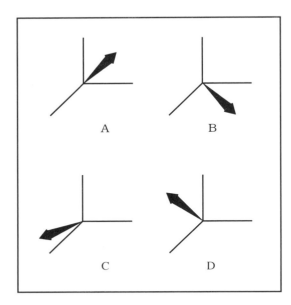

❑ **QUESTIONS TO PONDER**

13. When the patient is at equilibrium, where is M_0 with respect to the XYZ axes of the imager?

14. What does the vector arrow represent?

Worksheet | 21

RF Pulses

1. Two basic properties of a hydrogen nucleus important to MRI are:

   a. precession and mass
   b. mass and charge
   c. charge and spin
   d. spin and magnetic moment

2. When tissue is placed in a static magnetic field, the hydrogen nuclei tend to:

   a. spin with the field
   b. spin against the field
   c. align with the field
   d. align perpendicular to the field

3. Because the proton spins, it:

   a. relaxes
   b. induces
   c. has a magnetic moment
   d. has a precession

4. Because the proton spins, it will:

   a. invert   c. induce
   b. precess   d. relax

5. Net magnetization is the result of _____ of individual spins.

   a. the sum   c. the precession
   b. the difference d. the relaxation

6. At equilibrium, the net magnetization:

   a. is stationary   c. inverts
   b. precesses   d. relaxes

7. Which of the above vector diagrams represents a 360° RF pulse?

   a. A   c. C
   b. B   d. D

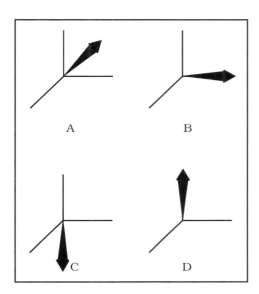

8. Which of the following contributes to the magnitude of M_0?

   a. T1 relaxation time   c. M_0
   b. T2 relaxation time   d. RF pulse

9. M_0 increases as _____ increases?

   a. spin density   c. T2 relaxation time
   b. T1 relaxation time   d. RF pulse

10. At equilibrium, no signal can be received from a patient because:

    a. B_0 is constant
    b. spin density is constant
    c. there is no M_{xy} component
    d. there is no M_z component

11. An RF pulse causes individual spins to:

    a. release energy and precess out of phase
    b. release energy and precess in phase
    c. absorb energy and precess out of phase
    d. absorb energy and precess in phase

12. An RF pulse causes the net magnetization to:

    a. shrink   c. disappear
    b. grow   d. flip

13. The degree of flip angle is determined by what characteristics of the RF pulse?

    a. time and precession
    b. precession and phase
    c. phase and intensity
    d. intensity and time

14. Short, intense RF pulses are called:

    a. hard pulses   c. round pulses
    b. soft pulses   d. square pulses

15. Low intensity, long RF pulses are called:

    a. hard pulses   c. round pulses
    b. soft pulses   d. square pulses

16. Which of the following vector diagrams represents a 90^0 RF pulse?

    a. A   c. C
    b. B   d. D

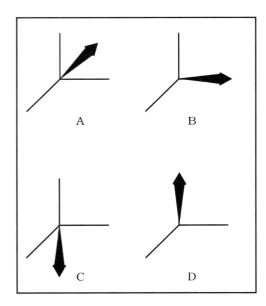

17. For a 20^0 flip angle:

    a. M_z shrinks as much as M_{xy}
    b. M_z shrinks more than M_{xy} shrinks
    c. M_z shrinks more than M_{xy} grows
    d. M_z shrinks less than M_{xy} grows

18. Following an alpha pulse:

    a. M_z and M_{xy} shrink
    b. M_z shrinks and M_{xy} grows
    c. M_z grows and M_{xy} shrinks
    d. M_z and M_{xy} grow

19. Following, which flip angle would the spin ensemble be saturated?

    a. 90^0 c. 360^0
    b. 180^0 d. alpha

20. Which of the vector diagrams in the preceding illustration represents a 20^0 RF pulse?

    a. A   c. C
    b. B   d. D

21. Following a 90^0 RF pulse, the net magnetization vector precesses because individual spins:

    a. precess in phase
    b. precess out of phase
    c. are partially saturated
    d. are at equilibrium

22. Following a 90^0 RF pulse, changes in M_z and M_{xy} are:

    a. dependent on B_0
    b. dependent on M_0
    c. dependent on each other
    d. independent of each other

23. Following a 90^0 RF pulse, M_z :

    a. remains at 0   c. remains at M_0
    b. relaxes to M_0 d. relaxes to 0

24. Following a 90^0 RF pulse, M_{xy}:

    a. remains at 0   c. remains at M_0
    b. relaxes to M_0 d. relaxes to 0

25. Following a 180^0 RF pulse, M_z:

    a. remains at 0   c. remains at M_0
    b. relaxes to M_0 d. relaxes to 0

26. Following a 180° RF pulse, M_{xy}:

    a. remains at 0   c. remains at M_0
    b. relaxes to M_0 d. relaxes to 0

27. Following an alpha RF pulse:

    a. M_z changes more rapidly than M_{xy}
    b. M_z and M_{xy} change at the same rate
    c. M_z changes more slowly than M_{xy}
    d. the change in M_z is dependent upon the value of M_{xy}

28. Following a 90° RF pulse, the receiving antennae will detect the relaxation of:

    a. the M_z component
    b. the M_{xy} component
    c. M_z plus M_{xy}
    d. M_z minus M_{xy}

29. Which of the following vector diagrams represents a 180° RF pulse?

    a. A   c. C
    b. B   d. D

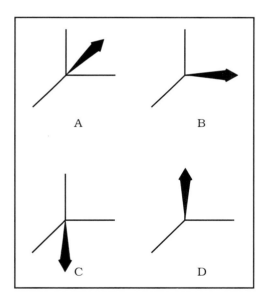

▢ **QUESTIONS TO PONDER**

30. Why must there be a range of frequencies in the RF pulse rather than a single frequency?

31. What does bandwidth (BW) relate to?

32. How long is the RF energized as a pulse?

33. What is "cross talk" and how is it avoided?

34. What method is employed to keep the spins saturated?

Worksheet

22

Spin Density

1. Which of the following is not a principle MRI parameter?

   a. Larmor frequency   c. T1 relaxation time
   b. spin density   d. T2 relaxation time

2. Tissue B has higher spin density than tissue A. Tissue B will:

   a. appear brighter
   b. appear darker
   c. have longer relaxation times
   d. have shorter relaxation times

3. Which of the following tissues should appear brightest, based strictly on spin density?

   a. fat   c. muscle
   b. water   d. bone

4. Which of the following tissues, based strictly on spin density should appear the darkest?

   a. fat   c. muscle
   b. water   d. bone

5. In addition to spin density, signal intensity is also affected by:

   a. how the spin is chemically bound
   b. how the spin is charged
   c. the mass of the spin
   d. the distribution of the spin

6. Spin density is most closely related to:

   a. bound hydrogen
   b. mobile hydrogen
   c. transient hydrogen
   d. induced hydrogen

7. Spin density can best be defined as hydrogen:

   a. concentration   c. relaxation
   b. charge   d. configuration

8. Spin density can best be described as the number of hydrogen nuclei:

   a. passing through a voxel
   b. at equilibrium in a voxel
   c. excited in a voxel
   d. in a voxel

9. Spin density is closest to the concentration of nuclei in:

   a. bound hydrogen   c. tissue
   b. mobile hydrogen   d. water

10. Spin density is most closely related to:

    a. precession   c. induction
    b. relaxation   d. concentration

11. Net magnetization at equilibrium (M_0) is most closely related to:

    a. spin density
    b. T1 relaxation time
    c. T2 relaxation time
    d. precession

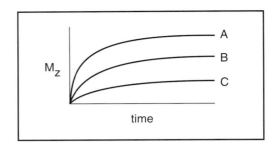

12. Which of the tissues represented in the above figure has the highest spin density?

    a. A
    b. B
    c. C
    d. not enough information

13. Which of the tissues represented in the above figure has the longest T1 relaxation time?

    a. A
    b. B
    c. C
    d. not enough information

14. Which of the tissues represented in the above figure has the longest T2 relaxation time?

    a. A
    b. B
    c. C
    d. not enough information

15. At equilibrium, M_z equals:

    a. M_o
    b. M_{xy}
    c. spin density
    d. relaxation

16. At equilibrium, M_z is undetectable because:

    a. it relaxes too fast
    b. the spin density is too low
    c. M_o is too high
    d. B_o is too high

17. The following figure is a graph of:

    a. spin density
    b. spin density relaxation
    c. longitudinal relaxation
    d. transverse relaxation

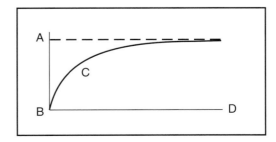

18. Spin density is most closely associated with a point at (refer to the bottom left figure):

    a. A
    b. B
    c. C
    d. D

19. The following figure is a graph of:

    a. spin density
    b. spin density relaxation
    c. longitudinal relaxation
    d. transverse relaxation

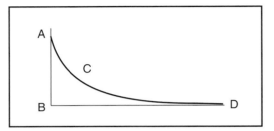

20. Spin density is most closely associated with a point at (refer to the above figure):

    a. A
    b. B
    c. C
    d. D

21. Arrange the following tissues according to their relative spin density (lowest spin density first).

    a. white matter   _____
    b. gray matter   _____
    c. blood   _____
    d. bone   _____

☐ QUESTIONS TO PONDER

22. What is the most important MR element in the body?

23. How is cartilage visualized in an image?

24. Does mAs in radiography have an MRI analog?

25. What is spin density (SD)?

26. How does spin density (SD) affect contrast?

Worksheet | 23 |

T1 Relaxation Time

1. T1 relaxation time is also known as:

    a. spin density
    b. longitudinal relaxation
    c. transverse relaxation
    d. precession

2. T1 relaxation occurs:

    a. rapidly at first, then slows down
    b. is constant
    c. slowly at first, then speeds up
    d. is discontinuous

3. T1 relaxation time is related to the time required for:

    a. M_z to return to equilibrium
    b. M_{xy} to return to equilibrium
    c. transverse saturation
    d. longitudinal saturation

4. The T1 relaxation time is 300 ms. What will be the value of M_z after a patient has been in a static magnetic field for 300 ms?

    a. 0.37 M_z c. 0.37 M_0
    b. 0.63 M_z d. 0.63 M_0

5. Which of the tissues in the following figure has the highest spin density?

    a. A   c. C
    b. B   d. not enough information

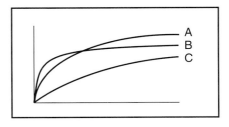

6. The T1 relaxation time for a given tissue is 600 ms. Upon removal from a magnet, what will be the value of M_z after 600 ms?

    a. 0.37 M_z c. 0.37 M_0
    b. 0.63 M_z d. 0.63 M_0

7. A given tissue has a T1 relaxation time of 750 ms. When a patient has been out of the magnet for 1.5 seconds, what will be the value of M_z?

    a. 0.37 M_z c. 0.37 M_0
    b. 0.14 M_z d. 0.14 M_0

8. T1 relaxation times are generally:

    a. shorter than T2 relaxation times
    b. about the same as T2 relaxation times
    c. longer than T2 relaxation times
    d. vary from tissue to tissue in relation to T2 relaxation times

9. After removal from the magnet for approximately five T1 relaxation times, M_z will equal approximately:

    a. 0   c. .63 M_0
    b. .37 M_0 d. M_0

10. Which of the following tissues has the longest T1 relaxation time?

    a. fat
    b. brain
    c. cerebral spinal fluid
    d. muscle

11. The time constant for the return of M_z to M_0 is:

    a. spin density
    b. T1 relaxation time
    c. T2 relaxation time
    d. precessional frequency

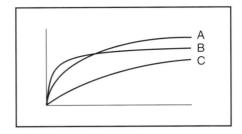

12. Which of the tissues in the above figure has the shortest T2 relaxation time?

    a. A
    b. B
    c. C
    d. not enough information

13. In general, as one increases B_0, the T1 relaxation time will:

    a. decrease
    b. remain the same
    c. increase
    d. vary from tissue to tissue

14. When M_z equals 0, it takes approximately _____ T1 relaxation times to return to equilibrium?

    a. 1
    b. 3
    c. 5
    d. 7

15. The term longitudinal, in longitudinal relaxation time refers to events occuring along the axis of the:

    a. patient
    b. static magnetic field
    c. magnetic field gradient
    d. radio antennae

16. Following an RF pulse, M_z will return to M_0, with a relaxation time described as:

    a. precessional
    b. inductional
    c. longitudinal
    d. transverse

17. Following an RF pulse, the return of M_z to M_0 is termed relaxation to:

    a. actuation
    b. saturation
    c. elongation
    d. equilibrium

18. Relaxation to equilibrium represents return to:

    a. a lower energy state
    b. the same energy state
    c. a higher energy state
    d. an energy state that is tissue dependent

19. In the term, spin lattice relaxation time, lattice refers to:

    a. stepping through T1, 2 T1, 3 T1. . .
    b. the spin quantum number of hydrogen
    c. the electron configuration of hydrogen
    d. the molecule in which the hydrogen is bound

20. During the return to equilibrium, spins give up energy to:

    a. other spins
    b. electrons
    c. the molecule
    d. the tissue

21. Generally, the appearance of tissue having a short T1 relaxation time on a T1 weighted image will appear:

    a. dark
    b. gray
    c. bright
    d. varies with tissue type

22. Which of the tissues in the preceding illustration has the shortest T1 relaxation time?

    a. A
    b. B
    c. C
    d. not enough information

23. In general, the T1 relaxation time:

    a. is shorter for diseased tissue
    b. is longer for diseased tissue.
    c. remains unchanged for diseased tissue
    d. is longer for some diseased tissues, shorter for others

24. The T1 relaxation time for a given tissue is 400 ms. What will be the value of M_z when a patient has been in a magnet for 800 ms?

    a. $0.63\ M_z$
    b. $0.86\ M_z$
    c. $0.63\ M_0$
    d. $0.86\ M_0$

☐ QUESTIONS TO PONDER

25. What are the three intrinsic MRI parameters?

26. What does lattice refer to in spin-lattice relaxation?

27. Approximately how much time is required for return to equilibrium following an RF pulse?

28. What unit is used for relaxation times?

29. When does T1 = T2?

Worksheet 24

T2 Relaxation Time

1. Transverse magnetization is symbolized by:

   a. B_0
   b. M_0
   c. M_{xy}
   d. M_z

2. Relaxation of transverse magnetization is controlled by:

   a. spin density
   b. T1 relaxation
   c. T2 relaxation
   d. precession

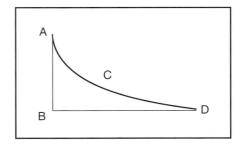

3. Which point in the above figure represents complete relaxation?

   a. A
   b. B
   c. C
   d. D

4. Relative to T1 relaxation times, T2 relaxation times are:

   a. very much shorter
   b. just a little shorter
   c. about the same
   d. a little bit longer

5. An FID is a result of relaxation of:

   a. B_0
   b. M_0
   c. M_{xy}
   d. M_z

6. The relaxation of M_z and M_{xy} are:

   a. interdependent only during early relaxation
   b. interdependent only during late relaxation
   c. interdependent
   d. independent

7. The term envelope of an FID refers to the:

   a. total relaxation time
   b. initial spin density
   c. length the signal is straightened
   d. line joining signal peaks

8. The figure below represents:

   a. spin density
   b. spin density relaxation
   c. T1 relaxation
   d. T2 relaxation

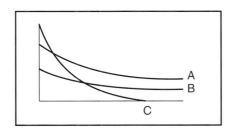

9. If B_0 were perfectly uniform, an FID would have an envelope described by:

   a. T1
   b. T1*
   c. T2
   d. T2*

10. On a T2-weighted image, tissues having:

   a. high spin density will appear dark
   b. high B_0 will appear bright
   c. short T2 will appear bright
   d. long T2 will appear bright

61

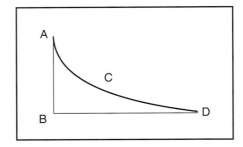

11. Referring to the T2 relaxation curve in the figure above, which point represents M_0?

    a. A   c. C
    b. B   d. D

12. When transverse magnetization relaxes, it returns to:

    a. 0   c. M_{xy}
    b. M_0 d. M_z

13. Which point in the figure above represents 0.37 M_0?

    a. A   c. C
    b. B   d. D

14. The regrowth of M_z to M_0 is a relaxation from:

    a. an excited state to equilibrium
    b. an excited state to zero
    c. zero to equilibrium
    d. equilibrium to an excited state

15. T2 relaxation is sometimes called _____ relaxation.

    a. spin-spin   c. equilibrium
    b. spin-lattice   d. precessional

16. Spin-spin relaxation represents relaxation:

    a. along the X axis   c. along the Z axis
    b. along the Y axis   d. in the XY plane

17. Transverse relaxation occurs in the _____ plane.

    a. XY   c. YZ
    b. XZ   d. ZO

18. Transverse relaxation occurs because:

    a. energy is absorbed from RF
    b. energy is released by RF
    c. spins exist separately
    d. spins interact with each other

19. Which of the following tissues is likely to have the longest T2 relaxation time?

    a. fat   c. CSF
    b. brain   d. muscle

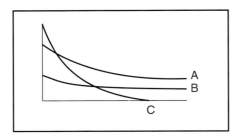

20. Which tissue in the figure above has the highest spin density?

    a. A   c. C
    b. B   d. not enough information

21. An FID demonstrates relaxation with a:

    a. time shorter than T2
    b. time equal to T2
    c. time longer than T2
    d. constant T2

22. T2* is:

    a. shorter than T2
    b. equal to T2
    c. longer than T2
    d. varies with tissue type

23. Spins that precess at the same frequency while pointing in different directions are said to be:

    a. in phase   c. at equilibrium
    b. out of phase   d. saturated

24. Spins that precess at the same frequency, all pointing at the same direction are said to be:

    a. in phase   c. at equilibrium
    b. out of phase   d. saturated

❒ QUESTIONS TO PONDER

25. How do SDW and T2W images often differ?

26. What is T2*?

27. Does tissue inhomogeneity increase or decrease spin dephasing?

28. How does varying B_0 affect T2?

How to Measure T2

1. Which of the following can be measured by direct observation?
   (1) time
   (2) distance
   (3) mass
   (4) relaxation time

   a. 1, 2, and 3   c. 2 and 4
   b. 1 and 3   d. 4

2. The FID does not represent true T2 relaxation time because of:

   a. different tissues within the same voxel
   b. magnetic susceptibility effects
   c. magnetic field inhomogeneity
   d. spin density inhomogeneity

3. The first half of a spin echo appears as:

   a. an FID
   b. the mirror image of an FID
   c. a 90⁰ RF pulse
   d. a 180⁰ RF pulse

4. How many FIDs are shown in the following figure?

   a. one   c. three
   b. two   d. four

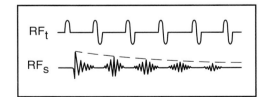

5. Determining T2 relaxation time is analogous to determining:

   a. radioactive half-life
   b. the time between two events
   c. the distance between two locations
   d. one's weight

6. Which of the following must be measured by computation following multiple observations ?
   (1) time
   (2) relaxation time
   (3) distance
   (4) radioactive decay

   a. 1, 2, and 3   c. 2 and 4
   b. 1 and 3   d. 4

7. Dephasing of spins within a region containing the same tissue occurs because of:
   (1) T1 relaxation
   (2) T2 relaxation
   (3) spin density inhomogeniety
   (4) magnetic field inhomogeneity

   a. 1, 2, and 3   c. 2 and 4
   b. 1 and 3   d. 4

8. The maximum amplitude of a spin echo occurs:

   a. at the beginning of the signal
   b. at the end of the signal
   c. at the midpoint of the signal
   d. variously according to pulse sequence

9. How many spin echoes are shown in the figure to the left?

   a. one   c. three
   b. two   d. four

10. The envelope of an FID is related to:

    a. T1   c. T1*
    b. T2   d. T2*

11 When nuclear spins dephase they:

    a. precess at slightly different frequencies
    b. precess at the same frequency
    c. change orientation with the external magnetic field
    d. transfer energy to the magnetic field

12. Echo time (TE) is the time:

    a. between the 90^0 RF pulse and the 180^0 RF pulse
    b. between the 90^0 RF pulse and the spin echo
    c. between the 180^0 RF pulse and the 90^0 RF pulse
    d. between the 180^0 RF pulse and the spin echo

13. T2 relaxation time is related to (refer to the figure below):

    a. A   c. C
    b. B   d. D

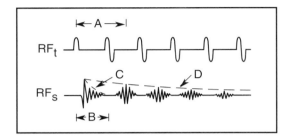

14. Which of the following relationships is correct?

    a. T1 is less than T1*
    b. T1 is greater than T1*
    c. T2 is less than T2*
    d. T2 is greater than T2*

15. In a spin echo pulse sequence nuclear spins are caused to rephase by:

    a. a 90^0 RF pulse
    b. a 180^0 RF pulse
    c. a change from T1 to T2 relaxation
    d. a change from T2 to T1 relaxation

16. As echo time increases, the amplitude of the spin echo:

    a. decreases
    b. remains constant
    c. increases
    d. depends on T1 relaxation time

17. In the figure to the left, T2* relaxation time is related to:

    a. A   c. C
    b. B   d. D

18. A spin echo is produced when:

    a. a 90^0 RF pulse is followed by a 180^0 RF pulse
    b. a 90^0 RF pulse is followed by a 90^0 RF pulse
    c. a 180^0 RF pulse is followed by a 90^0 RF pulse
    b. a 180^0 RF pulse is followed by a 180^0 RF pulse

19. Which of the following relationships is true?
    (1) 90^0 RF pulse to 180^0 RF pulse = 180^0 RF pulse to 90^0 RF pulse
    (2) 90^0 RF pulse to 180^0 RF pulse = 180^0 RF pulse to spin echo
    (3) 90^0 RF pulse to 180^0 RF pulse = echo time
    (4) 90^0 RF pulse to echo = echo time

    a. 1, 2, and 3   c. 2 and 4
    b. 1 and 3   d. 4

20. The amplitude of a spin echo is dependent on:
    (1) T1 relaxation time
    (2) T2 relaxation time
    (3) T2* relaxation time
    (4) echo time

    a. 1, 2, and 3   c. 2 and 4
    b. 1 and 3   d. 4

☐ **QUESTIONS TO PONDER**

21. What is the temporal relationship between T1 and T2 relaxation times?

22. Where is the TE set to obtain optimum tissue contrast?

23. Why is T2* relaxation time always shorter than T2?

24. Describe the graphic relationship between T2 and T2*.

Worksheet 26

How to Measure T1

1. T1 relaxation occurs:

    a. along the X axis   c. in the XY plane
    b. along the Y axis   d. along the Z axis

2. In order to measure M_z one must use the following pulse sequence:

    a. 90^0...90^0 c. 180^0...90^0
    b. 90^0...180^0 d. 180^0...180^0

3. As the inversion delay time (TI) is increased :

    a. the amplitude of the FID increases
    b. the amplitude of the FID decreases
    c. T1 relaxation time increases
    d. T2 relaxation time increases

4. Which of the diagrams in the following figure can best be used to estimate T1 relaxation time?

    a. A   c. C
    b. B   d. D

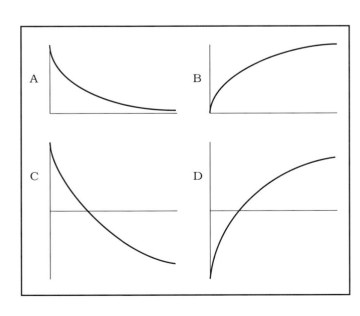

5. Magnetization of tissue along the Z axis cannot be measured directly because:
    (1) the B_0 field is too intense
    (2) M_{xy} is too small
    (3) M_z is too small
    (4) T1 relaxation time is too short

    a. 1, 2, and 3   c. 2 and 4
    b. 1 and 3   d. 4

6. M_z can only be measured by flipping magnetization:

    a. back to equilibrium
    b. to the +Z direction axis
    c. onto the XY plane
    d. to the -Z direction

7. Following a very long inversion delay time:
    (1) T1 relaxation time will be very long
    (2) T2 relaxation time will be very long
    (3) the FID will be very strong
    (4) the FID will be very weak

    a. 1, 2, and 3   c. 2 and 4
    b. 1 and 3   d. 4

8. The inversion delay time (TI) is the time between the:

    a. 90^0 RF pulse and 90^0 RF pulse
    b. 90^0 RF pulse and 180^0 RF pulse
    c. 180^0 RF pulse and 90^0 RF pulse
    d. 180^0 RF pulse and 180^0 RF pulse

9. T1 relaxation time can be measured:
    (1) indirectly
    (2) from multiple spin echoes
    (3) from multiple FIDs
    (4) from a single FID

    a. 1, 2, and 3   c. 2 and 4
    b. 1 and 3   d. 4

10. Following a 180^0 RF pulse:

   a. $M_z = -M_0$
   b. $M_z = 0$

   c. $M_z = M_0$
   d. $M_z = M_{xy}$

11. Following an inversion recovery pulse sequence:
   (1) an FID is observed
   (2) a spin echo is observed
   (3) spin magnetization is in the XY plane
   (4) spin magnetization is along the Z axis

   a. 1, 2, and 3
   b. 1 and 3

   c. 2 and 4
   d. 4

12. The time necessary to measure T1:

   a. is less than than required for T2 determination
   b. is about the same as that required for T2 determination
   c. is much longer than that required for T2 determination
   d. depends on the spin echo pulse sequence employed

13. The figure below is a graph of:

   a. spin density
   b. spin density relaxation
   c. longitudinal relaxation
   d. transverse relaxation

14. Which tissue in the figure below has the highest spin density?

   a. A
   b. B

   c. C
   d. not enough information

15. Which tissue in the figure below has the shortest T1 relaxation time?

   a. A
   b. B

   c. C
   d. not enough information

16. Which tissue in the following figure has the shortest T2 relaxation time?

   a. A
   b. B

   c. C
   d. not enough information

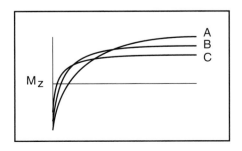

□ QUESTIONS TO PONDER

17. Compare T1 relaxation to T2 relaxation.

18. What is a signal envelope?

19. What does T1 ≥ T2 mean?

20. How does varying B_0 affect T1?

21. Does increased signal amplitude always produce a brighter image?

Worksheet 27

Nuclear Species

1. The term spectrum is also referred to as:

   a. precession
   b. relaxation time
   c. frequency distribution
   d. nuclear species

2. A spectrum is usually a graph of intensity as a function of:

   a. mass
   b. frequency
   c. electric potential
   d. relaxation time

3. An NMR spectrum is a plot of:

   a. signal intensity vs frequency
   b. signal intensity vs wave length
   c. frequency vs time
   d. wave length vs time

4. An NMR spectrum is obtained from:

   a. spin density
   b. relaxation time
   c. magnetic field gradient
   d. free induction decay

5. The NMR spectrum is obtain from an MR signal through the process of:

   a. Fourier transformation
   b. signal relaxation
   c. back projection reconstruction
   d. complex restoration

6. When one Fourier transforms an MR signal, one obtains a distribution of intensity as a function of:

   a. mass
   b. time
   c. inverse time
   d. spin density

7. Which nuclear species would show the highest signal intensity from an NMR spectrum of the human body?

   a. hydrogen
   b. nitrogen
   c. oxygen
   d. carbon

8. Which of the following medically important nuclei has the highest gyromagnetic ratio?

   a. hydrogen
   b. nitrogen
   c. oxygen
   d. carbon

9. A nuclear species such as oxygen-16, which has a spin quantum number of zero, most likely has a gyromagnetic ratio near:

   a. 0 MHz/T
   b. 10 MHz/T
   c. 20 MHz/T
   d. 40 MHz/T

10. Which of the hydrogen peaks in the following figure represents a chemical shift of 10 ppm in a 1 T magnet?

    a. A
    b. B
    c. C
    d. D

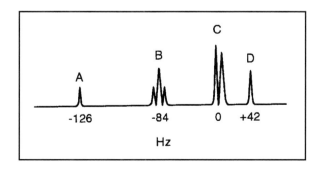

11. The hydrogen spectrum of tissue is dominated by:

    a. water and fat   c. fat and muscle
    b. water and muscle   d. muscle and bone

12. The most prominent peak in the hydrogen spectrum of tissue is due to:

    a. fat   c. muscle
    b. water   d. bone

13. The Larmor frequency of hydrogen in water is:

    a. lower than that for fat
    b. equal to that for fat
    c. higher than that for fat
    d. independent of field strength

14. The separation of the Larmor frequency between water and fat, when imaging tissue is:

    a. 42 ppm   c. 225 ppm
    b. 100 ppm   d. 1000 ppm

15. The chemical shift between water and fat at 0.5 tesla is 225 ppm. The shift at 1.5 tesla will be:

    a. 112.5 ppm   c. 450 ppm
    b. 225 ppm   d. 675 ppm

16. Chemical shift artifacts usually show up at:

    a. low magnetic field strength
    b. intermediate magnetic field strength
    c. high magnetic field strength
    d. all magnetic field strength

17. The principle peak in a phosphorous NMR spectrum is due to:

    a. alpha ATP   c. gamma ATP
    b. beta ATP   d. creatine phosphate

18. Phosphorous shows promise for in vivo NMR because it is an active metabolite. The nuclear species involved is:

    a. P-30   c. P-32
    b. P-31   d. P-33

19. The carbon nucleus investigated for in vivo NMR spectroscopy is:

    a. C-10   c. C-12
    b. C-11   d. C-13

20. The fluorine nucleus being investigated for in vivo NMR is:

    a. F-17   c. F-19
    b. F-18   d. F-20

21. The NMR spectrum of hydrogen does not contain information about phosphorous because of differences in:

    a. spin density
    b. relaxation times
    c. nuclear mass
    d. Larmor frequency

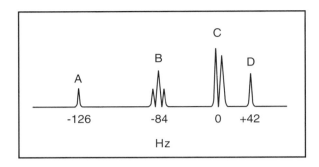

22. Which of the hydrogen peaks in the above figure represents a chemical shift of 30 ppm in a 1 T magnet?

    a. A   c. C
    b. B   d. D

☐ QUESTIONS TO PONDER

23. Describe a hydrogen atom and a water molecule.

24. Why don't all nuclei respond equally to B_0?

25. What is the relationship between peak separation and magnetic field strength in magnetic resonance spectroscopy?

Worksheet | **28**

Chemical Shift

1. The term chemical shift relates principally to a change in:

   a. spin density   c. nuclear mass
   b. relaxation times   d. Larmor frequency

2. A nuclear species may exhibit more than one peak in an NMR spectrum because of its:

   a. nuclear structure
   b. electron configuration
   c. molecular configuration
   d. mass distribution

3. The NMR spectrum is related to _____ structure.

   a. nuclear   c. molecular
   b. electron shell   d. organ

4. A hydrogen NMR spectrum may have many peaks because each nucleus has slightly different:

   a. spin density   c. nuclear mass
   b. relaxation time   d. Larmor frequency

5. The change in resonant frequency among similar atoms in the same molecule is due to slight changes in:

   a. the static magnetic field
   b. spin density
   c. relaxation times
   d. the local magnetic field

6. A change in resonant frequency for similar atoms in a given molecule is caused by:

   a. spin density   c. electron cloud
   b. relaxation times   d. nuclear structure

7. If an NMR spectrum contained just two peaks, that would indicate two:

   a. spin densities   c. different nuclei
   b. relaxation times   d. types of bound atoms

8. The more peaks there are in an NMR spectrum, the more different types of _____ there will be.

   a. nuclear configurations
   b. bound nuclei
   c. nuclear species
   d. nuclear relaxation

9. The shift or separation of peaks in an NMR spectrum increases with increasing:

   a. spin density   c. gyromagnetic ratio
   b. relaxation time   d. B_0

10. The finest separation of peaks in an NMR spectrum will be obtained at _____ magnetic field strength.

    a. high   c. low
    b. intermediate   d. variable

11. The Larmor frequency for hydrogen at 0.5 T is 21 MHz. A second peak is observed at a separation of 100 parts per million. What is the equivalent frequency separation?

    a. 100 Hz   c. 2100 Hz
    b. 100 kHz   d. 2100 kHz

12. At 1 T, the hydrogen Larmor frequency is 42 MHz. A second peak occurs at 42.021 MHz. This chemical shift is equal to:

    a. 210 ppm   c. 21,000 ppm
    b. 500 ppm   d. 50,000 ppm

13. At 1.5 T, a hydrogen NMR spectrum exhibits peaks at 62.9999 MHz and 63.0002 MHz. This represents a chemical shift of:

    a. 63 ppm   c. 300 ppm
    b. 100 ppm   d. 999 ppm

14. At 1.0 T, a hydrogen chemical shift of 8 ppm is observed. This represents a frequency difference of:

    a. 42 ppm
    b. 84 ppm
    c. 336 ppm
    d. 500 ppm

15. At 0.5 T, a hydrogen NMR spectrum exhibits a chemical shift of 6 ppm. The chemical shift at 1.5 T will be:

    a. 2 ppm
    b. 6 ppm
    c. 18 ppm
    d. 27 ppm

16. A hydrogen NMR spectrum exhibits a chemical shift of 12 ppm at 1 T. At 0.5 T, the chemical shift will be:

    a. 63 Hz
    b. 126 Hz
    c. 252 Hz
    d. 504 Hz

17. A 1.0 T magnet is said to have homogeneity of ± 10 ppm. This represents:

    a. ±10 T
    b. ±10 mT
    c. ±10μT
    d. ±10 nT

18. A 0.3 T magnet has magnetic field homogeneity of ± 40 ppm. The range of resonant frequency for this magnet will be:

    a. ±.3 Hz
    b. ± 42 Hz
    c. ± 504 Hz
    d. ± 2,000 Hz

19. The number of uniquely bound nuclei in an NMR spectrum is related to:

    a. the number of peaks
    b. the area under the peaks
    c. the height of the peaks
    d. the parts per million

20. The fine structure contained in an individual peak of an NMR spectrum is due to:

    a. J-coupling
    b. M_0
    c. B_0
    d. R-coupling

21. J-coupling is independent of:

    a. B_0
    b. M_0
    c. SD
    d. T1 or T2

22. J-coupling is dependent on:

    a. M_0
    b. B_0
    c. nearby electrons
    d. nearby nuclei

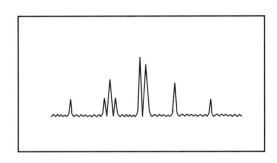

23. The above figure shows an NMR spectrum containing eight peaks of varying heights. The height of each is related to the:

    a. number of spins
    b. spin relaxation
    c. longitudinal relaxation
    d. transverse relaxation

24. In the ethanol spectrum, the number of peaks is related to the:

    a. spin quantum number
    b. different bonding of hydrogen
    c. different longitudinal relaxation
    d. different transverse relaxation

☐ QUESTIONS TO PONDER

25. What is chemical shift?

26. How is chemical shift measured?

27. What is tissue specificity?

28. How do the T1 and T2 relaxation times vary for unbound water and fat?

29. What is the chemical shift between fat and water at 4 T?

The Computer's View of the World

1. Match the following:
   (1) direct interaction with image receptor
   (2) induced electronic impulses
   (3) spatial frequency information
   (4) filtered back-projection reconstruction

   a. MRI image   _____
   b. X-ray image   _____
   c. ultrasound image   _____
   d. computed tomography image _____

2. MRI signals are obtained in the _____ and converted by Fourier transformation to the _____.

   a. Cartesian coordinates, polar coordinates
   b. frequency data, phase data
   c. spatial location domain, spatial frequency domain
   d. spatial frequency domain, spatial location domain

3. Any number raised to the 0 power, such as 13 will have a value of:

   a. 0   c. 13
   b. 1   d. 130

4. The number 234 can be expressed in binary fashion as:

   a. 01001111   c. 01101111
   b. 01010111   d. 01101001

5. A digital image with an 9 bit matrix size would have _____ pixels.

   a. 64 x 64   c. 256 x 256
   b. 128 x 128 d. 512 x 512

6. One kilobyte is equal to:

   a. 2^3 c. 2^{10}
   b. 2^6 d. 2^{20}

7. One gigabyte is equal to:

   a. 2^5 c. 2^{20}
   b. 2^{10} d. 2^{30}

8. The term precision when applied to MRI describes:
   (1) the exactness of a measurement
   (2) the number of values in a measurement
   (3) the ability to distinguish one small number from another
   (4) a continuous range of values

   a. 1, 2, and 3   c. 2 and 4
   b. 1 and 3   d. 4

9. The human visual system can resolve about _____ different shades of gray.

   a. 8   c. 128
   b. 32   d. 512

10. A good example of sampling a continuous signal is:

    a. the detection of an MRI signal
    b. the detection of a video signal
    c. the display of an MRI image
    d. the display of a video image

11. When sampling the MRI signal, the lower limit on the sampling rate is determined by:

    a. the capacity of the computer
    b. the strength of the MRI signal
    c. the spatial frequency range of the MRI signal
    d. the rate needed to avoid aliasing

12. The sonogram is an image obtained during:

    a. MRI   c. DSA
    b. CT   d. diagnostic ultrasound

13. Digital computers work with:

    a. alphanumerics   c. decimal values
    b. binary numbers d. bits, bites and chumps

14. When the dynamic range of an MR imager has 2^8 shades of gray, this is equivalent to _____ shades of gray.

    a. 2   c. 16
    b. 8   d. 256

15. The binary number 10101 is equal to:

    a. 15   c. 21
    b. 19   d. 27

16. An image having an 8 bit dynamic range would have _____ shades of gray.

    a. 8   c. 256
    b. 64   d. 512

17. One kilobyte is equal to:

    a. 100 bytes   c. 1024 bytes
    b. 1000 bytes   d. 2048 bytes

18. How many bits can be stored on a 2 megabyte chip:

    a. 2^{20} c. 2^{28}
    b. 2×2^{20} d. 2×2^{28}

19. Another term for dynamic range is:

    a. dynamic values
    b. gray values
    c. contrast resolution
    d. gray scale resolution

20. Limited dynamic range can result in:

    a. reduced signal to noise
    b. false contouring
    c. extended imaging time
    d. false relaxation times

21. MRI signals that change value very rapidly are said to have:

    a. slow relaxation times
    b. high fast relaxation times
    c. low frequency
    d. high frequency

22. When sampling an MRI signal, the upper limit on the rate is determined by the:

    a. capacity of the computer
    b. strength of the MRI signal
    c. spatial frequency range of the MRI signal
    d. rate needed to avoid aliasing

23. A sonogram presents data in the:

    a. spatial frequency domain
    b. spatial localization domain
    c. temporal location domain
    d. temporal induction domain

24. A single number used in the digital computer is a BIT, which stands for:

    a. big digit   c. binary toe
    b. big toe   d. binary digit

25. The number 131 can be expressed in binary fashion as:

    a. 11010010   c. 11000010
    b. 10101100   d. 10100110

26. The binary number 110011 may be expressed as:

    a. 39   c. 57
    b. 51   d. 63

27. To encode is to translate:
    (1) a decimal number to a binary number
    (2) a binary number to a decimal number
    (3) an alphabetic character to a binary number
    (4) an alphabetic character to a decimal number

    a. 1, 2, and 3   c. 2 and 4
    b. 1 and 3   d. all are correct

28. One megabyte is equal to:

    a. 2^3 c. 2^{10}
    b. 2^6 d. 2^{20}

29. How many bits can be stored on a 16 megabyte chip?

    a. 2^{10} bits   c. 2^{27} bits
    b. 2^{20} bits   d. 2^{30} bits

30. A large dynamic range is associated with:

    a. better contrast resolution
    b. better spatial resolution
    c. the number of different shades of gray
    d. reduced imaging time

31. The free induction decay is:

    a. a number of samples
    b. an exponential curve
    c. a discrete signal
    d. a continuous signal

32. When a rapidly changing MRI signal is not sampled frequently enough:

    a. the data becomes truncated
    b. the data becomes aliased
    c. spatial resolution is reduced
    d. contrast resolution is reduced

33. The MRI signal contains intensities which change value with:
    (1) time
    (2) charge
    (3) space
    (4) energy

    a. 1, 2, and 3   c. 2 and 4
    b. 1 and 3   d. 4

34. MRI signal data can be presented as both:

    a. x and y coordinated
    b. distance and angle values
    c. magnitude and phase
    d. frequency and phase

35. Binary digits can take on values of:

    a. 0 and 1   c. 0, 1 . . . 9
    b. 0, 1 . . . 5   d. 0, 1 . . . 99

36. The number 679 can be expressed in binary fashion as:

    a. 1100101101   c. 1110001101
    b. 1100110101   d. 1110010101

37. The binary number 1000111 is equal to:

    a. 63   c. 101
    b. 91   d. 113

38. One byte is equal to:

    a. 1 bit   c. 8 bits
    b. 2 bits   d. 16 bits

39. One megabyte is equal to:

    a. 1000 bytes   c. 1024 bytes
    b. 1,000,000 bytes d. 1,048,576 bytes

40. A 10-bit computer number can take on values of:

    a. 0 through 255   c. 0 through 1023
    b. 255 through 1023 d. 0 through 1024

41. The dynamic range of the human eye is somewhere between:

    a. 2^0 and 2^2 c. 2^4 and 2^6
    b. 2^2 and 2^4 d. 2^6 and 2^8

42. The term sampling, when applied to MRI relates to:

    a. detecting an MRI signal
    b. reconstruction and MRI image
    c. measuring the value of an MRI signal at regular intervals
    d. conducting a Fourier transform on the MRI signal

43. In order to avoid aliasing, the MRI signal must be sampled:

    a. continuously
    b. at least once in each signal direction
    c. at least twice in each signal direction
    d. at least three times in each signal direction

❒ QUESTIONS TO PONDER

44. What does encode mean?

45. Define signal-to-noise ratio (S/N).

46. How can S/N be increased?

47. Define field of view (FOV).

48. How does scan time change with a change in FOV?

Worksheet | 30 |

The Spatial Frequency Domain

1. Spatial resolution is normally measured in:
   (1) line pairs per centimeter
   (2) cycles per centimeter
   (3) line pairs per millimeter
   (4) cycles per millimeter

   a. 1, 2, and 3   c. 2 and 4
   b. 1 and 3   d. all are correct

2. The ability to image objects with low spatial frequencies, is the ability to image:

   a. very small objects
   b. very large objects
   c. low contrast objects
   d. high contrast objects

3. Rank the following ability to image from lowest spatial frequency objects to highest spatial frequency objects (lowest = 1).

   a. screen-film   _____
   b. the human eye   _____
   c. magnetic resonance imager _____
   d. image intensifier   _____

4. In general, the contrast resolution of an image will improve as the:
   (1) pixel size gets larger
   (2) the image matrix size gets larger
   (3) low spatial frequencies are adequately sampled
   (4) high spatial frequencies are adequately sampled

   a. 1, 2, and 3   c. 2 and 4
   b. 1 and 3   d. 4

5. The dynamic range of an MR image is described as 8 bits deep. How many bytes is required for each pixel?

   a. 1   c. 4
   b. 2   d. 8

6. One line pair per millimeter is equal to _____ line pair per centimeter.

   a. 0.01   c. 1.0
   b. 0.1   d. 10

7. Which of the following can image the smallest object?

   a. a radioisotope scan
   b. the human eye
   c. an image intensifier
   d. MRI

8. A high spatial frequency represents:
   (1) a very small object
   (2) rapid changes of the MRI signal
   (3) good spatial resolution
   (4) a short signal time

   a. 1, 2, and 3   c. 2 and 4
   b. 1 and 3   d. all are correct

9. In general, the signal to noise ratio of an image will improve as the:
   (1) pixel size gets smaller
   (2) the image matrix size gets larger
   (3) high spatial frequencies are adequately sampled
   (4) low spatial frequencies are adequately sampled

   a. 1, 2, and 3   c. 2 and 4
   b. 1 and 3   d. 4

10. A 2^8 x 2^8 image matrix is 8 bits deep. How many bytes for this image are required?

   a. 8   c. 65,536
   b. 64   d. 524,288

11. The ability to image objects with high spatial frequencies is the ability to image:

   a. very small objects
   b. very large objects
   c. low contrast objects
   d. high contrast objects

12. Which type of image can reproduce the highest frequency?

    a. diagnostic ultrasound
    b. magnetic resonance imaging
    c. computed tomography
    d. screen-film

13. An image matrix is a:

    a. rendering of tissue spin densities
    b. rendering of tissue relaxation times
    c. grid of cells or boxes containing numbers
    d. finite row of numbers

14. When an MRI image matrix is described as 512 x 512. It can also be described as:

    a. 2^3 x 2^3 c. 2^7 x 2^7
    b. 2^5 x 2^5 d. 2^9 x 2^9

15. The minimum matrix size that does not appear blocky is approximately:

    a. 8 x 8   c. 128 x 128
    b. 32 x 32   d. 512 x 512

16. Rank the following ability to image from lowest spatial frequency objects to highest spatial frequency objects (lowest = 1).

    a. diagnostic ultrasound   _____
    b. direct exposure film   _____
    c. computed tomography   _____
    d. radioisotope scan   _____

17. In general, the spatial resolution of an image will improve as the:
    (1) pixel size gets smaller
    (2) the image matrix size gets larger
    (3) high spatial frequencies are adequately sampled
    (4) low spatial frequencies are adequately sampled

    a. 1, 2, and 3   c. 2 and 4
    b. 1 and 3   d. 4

18. An MR image is reconstructed as a 2^6 x 2^6 image matrix. The image matrix is also:

    a. 64 x 64   c. 256 x 256
    b. 128 x 128   d. 512 x 512

19. The matrix size that does not appear blocky is approximately:

    a. 2^3 x 2^3 c. 2^7 x 2^7
    b. 2^5 x 2^5 d. 2^9 x 2^9

20. The spatial frequency domain is often identified as:

    a. A-space   c. T-space
    b. K-space   d. Z-space

21. An MRI signal contains a:

    a. direct visual pattern
    b. range of frequencies
    c. range of energies
    d. latent image

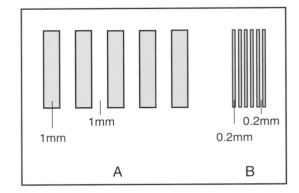

22. In the figure above, the spatial frequency of B:

    a. will relax faster than A
    b. represents higher spin density than A
    c. is higher than A
    d. represents larger objects than A

23. In the figure above, the spatial frequency of pattern B equals:

    a. 0.2 lp/mm   c. 2.5 lp/mm
    b. 0.4 lp/mm   d. 5 lp/mm

☐ **QUESTIONS TO PONDER**

24. How are contrast resolution, signal-to-noise ratio (S/N) and scan time affected by slice thickness?

25. Why is the term "echo" used?

26. What happens to spatial resolution and contrast resolution with an increase in field of view (FOV)?

27. Why does FOV affect image contrast?

Worksheet 31

Magnetic and RF Field Distortion Artifacts

1. A 1.0 T MR imager is said to have B_0 field homogeneity of ± 20 ppm. That is equivalent to:

   a. ± 2 microtesla   c. ± 2 millitesla
   b. ± 20 microtesla   d. ± 20 millitesla

2. Ferromagnetic material contains no hydrogen; therefore at that location:

   a. spin density is zero
   b. electron density is zero
   c. T1 relaxation time is increased
   d. T2 relaxation time is increased

3. The chemical shift artifact is usually:

   a. in the frequency encoding direction
   b. in the phase encoding direction
   c. throughout the slice selected
   d. along the RF axis

4. Using a 1.0 T imager the soft tissue/fat chemical shift artifact occurs because of a Larmor frequency difference of:

   a. 3.5 Hz   c. 75 Hz
   b. 35 Hz   d. 149 Hz

5. System-related field homogeneity artifacts may be caused by:
   (1) the X gradient coil
   (2) the Y gradient coil
   (3) the Z gradient coil
   (4) the B_0 coil

   a. 1, 2, and 3   c. 2 and 4
   b. 1 and 3   d. all are correct

6. An image artifact can best be described as:

   a. something left behind in the patient
   b. something absent in the patient
   c. an unwanted pattern that does not represent actual anatomy
   d. positive or negative enhancement of actual anatomy

7. A 0.5 T MR imager is said to have B_0 field homogeneity of ± 10 ppm. This is equal to:

   a. ± 0.5 microtesla   c. ± 50 microtesla
   b. ± 5 microtesla   d. ± 500 microtesla

8. Metal-induced artifacts in MR differ from those in CT in that:

   a. they are local in nature
   b. they result in streaking across the image
   c. they produce an increased mottling
   d. a herringbone pattern is visible

9. The chemical shift artifact is usually viewed as:

   a. streaking from an interface
   b. a herringbone pattern
   c. a bright or dark rim to an organ
   d. an increased mottled appearance

10. When using a 1.5 T imager, soft tissue/fat chemical shift artifact occursbecause of a Larmor frequency difference of:

    a. 35 Hz   c. 149 Hz
    b. 75 Hz   d. 224 Hz

11. Images that are particularly sensitive to magnetic field inhomogeneities are:
    (1) those produced by surface coils
    (2) those produced by the body coil
    (3) GRE images
    (4) spin echo images

    a. 1, 2, and 3   c. 2 and 4
    b. 1 and 3   d. all are correct

12. A useful scheme for classifying MRI artifacts would include:
    (1) magnetic field distortion artifacts
    (2) reconstruction artifacts
    (3) noise-induced artifacts
    (4) RF field distortion artifacts

    a. 1, 2, and 3   c. 2 and 4
    b. 1 and 3   d. all are correct

13. Distortion of B_0 magnetic field homogeneity can be caused by:
    (1) a poorly shimmed magnet
    (2) tissue magnetic susceptibility
    (3) ferromagnetic materials
    (4) a shift in the Larmor frequency

    a. 1, 2, and 3   c. 2 and 4
    b. 1 and 3   d. all are correct

14. Ferromagnetic objects distort the local magnetic field and therefore:

    a. change the spin density
    b. lengthen T1 relaxation time
    c. lengthen T2 relaxation time
    d. change the local Larmor frequency

15. The principal chemical shift artifact is that due to interfaces of:

    a. air and tissue   c. fat and bone
    b. fat and tissue   d. bone and air

16. The chemical shift artifact is visualized because the Larmor frequency shift causes tissue to:

    a. appear distorted   c. appear shifted
    b. appear mottled   d. shift

17. Any classification of MRI image artifacts can be categorized as:
    (1) spin density–related artifacts
    (2) patient-related artifacts
    (3) relaxation time–related artifacts
    (4) system-related artifacts

    a. 1, 2, and 3   c. 2 and 4
    b. 1 and 3   d. all are correct

18. Foreign ferromagnetic material in the patient can produce:
    (1) streaking artifacts
    (2) local signal loss
    (3) ring artifacts
    (4) warping distortion

    a. 1, 2, and 3   c. 2 and 4
    b. 1 and 3   d. all are correct

19. Inhomogeneities both in the B_0 field and the RF pulse can be caused by:
    (1) the patientís shape
    (2) the electrical conductivity of the patient
    (3) extension of the patient out of the imaging coil
    (4) the fat content of the patient

    a. 1, 2, and 3   c. 2 and 4
    b. 1 and 3   d. all are correct

20. The figure below (courtesy Errol Candy, Dallas) shows:

    a. a chemical shift artifact
    b. a field inhomogeneity artifact
    c. a truncation artifact
    d. ghosting because of CSF pulsation

21. The phase encoding gradient was applied along the:

    a. X axis   c. Z axis
    b. Y axis   d. can't tell

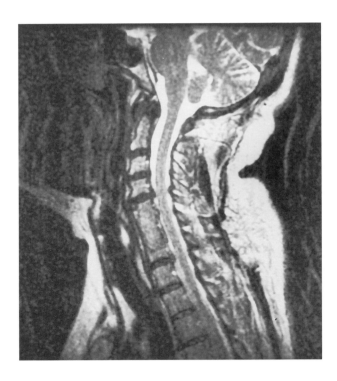

❏ QUESTIONS TO PONDER

22. What is an image artifact?

23. Which image axis is associated with chemical shift artifacts?

Worksheet | 32

Reconstruction Artifacts

1. The partial volume averaging artifact can be reduced by:

    a. obtaining more signal averages
    b. increasing TR
    c. reducing flip angle
    d. reducing slice thickness

2. The truncation artifact is more pronounced when the:

    a. repetition time is long
    b. repetition time is short
    c. number of phase encoding acquisitions is large
    d. number of phase encoding acquisitions is small

3. The quadrature detection artifact occurs along the:

    a. transverse axis
    b. longitudinal axis
    c. phase encoding axis
    d. frequency encoding axis

4. Which of the following would be considered a reconstruction artifact?
    (1) aliasing
    (2) partial volume averaging
    (3) truncation
    (4) quadrature defects

    a. 1, 2, and 3   c. 2 and 4
    b. 1 and 3   d. all are correct

5. The partial volume averaging artifact exists when:

    a. a structure is not fully contained within a slice
    b. a structure is contained within three or more slices
    c. the repetition time is too short
    d. the repetition time is too long

6. The truncation artifact can:
    (1) be along the frequency encoding axis
    (2) be along the phase encoding axis
    (3) result from a small reconstruction matrix
    (4) result from improper repetition time

    a. 1, 2, and 3   c. 2 and 4
    b. 1 and 3   d. all are correct

7. The aliasing artifact occurs when:

    a. using an improper RF pulse sequence
    b. using incorrect magnetic field gradients
    c. RF excited tissue is outside the field of view
    d. RF excitation of tissue is not uniform

8. To truncate is to:

    a. reshape an object
    b. lop off part of the object
    c. stretch an object
    d. slice an object

9. The quadrature detection artifact is sometimes called:

    a. ringing artifact
    b. zipper artifact
    c. herringbone artifact
    d. wraparound artifact

10. The aliasing artifact is sometimes identified as:

    a. Gibbs' phenomena
    b. wraparound artifact
    c. frequency-phase artifact
    d. conehead artifact

11. The truncation artifact is sometimes referred to as:

    a. wraparound artifact
    b. ringing artifact
    c. Gibbs' phenomena
    d. herringbone effect

12. The quadrature detection artifact occurs because of a problem with the:

    a. B_0 magnetic field
    b. gradient magnetic field
    c. RF system
    d. patient characteristics

13. The aliasing artifact is always:

    a. related to spin density differences
    b. related to relaxation time differences
    c. along the frequency-encoding direction
    d. along the phase-encoding direction

14. The truncation artifact appears as:

    a. a herringbone pattern
    b. increased mottle
    c. multiple curve lines
    d. streaks off a bony prominence

❒ QUESTIONS TO PONDER

15. Define aliasing.

16. How can aliasing be eliminated?

17. How can truncation be reduced?

18. How does matrix size vary with a change in field of view (FOV)?

19. What happens to image quality when a small clinical area is magnified?

SECTION II

Data Acquisition and Processing

Worksheet | 33 |

RF Pulse Sequences

1. Following a 90° RF pulse, the signal received from the patient is:

   a. none
   b. a free induction decay
   c. a spin echo
   d. a gradient-refocused echo

2. Following a 180° RF pulse, the signal received from the patient is:

   a. none
   b. a free induction decay
   c. a spin echo
   d. a gradient-refocused echo

3. Following a 270° RF pulse, the signal received from the patient is:

   a. none
   b. a free induction decay
   c. a spin echo
   d. a gradient-refocused echo

4. The symbol for a zero degree RF pulse is (refer to the figure below):

   a. A   c. C
   b. B   d. D

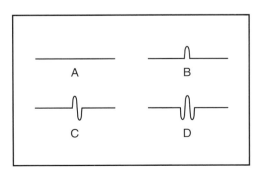

5. The symbol for an alpha RF pulse is (refer to the preceding figure):

   a. A   c. C
   b. B   d. D

6. The symbol for a 90° RF pulse is (refer to the preceding figure):

   a. A   c. C
   b. B   d. D

7. The symbol for 180° RF pulse is (refer to the preceding figure):

   a. A   c. C
   b. B   d. D

8. The initial amplitude of an FID is dependent of all but which one of the following?

   a. relaxation time   c. B_0
   b. spin density   d. gyromagnetic ratio

9. FIDs are not used for imaging, principally because:

   a. they are too weak
   b. they are too strong
   c. of magnet engineering demands
   d. of antennae engineering demands

10. The term pulse sequence refers to:

    a. RF pulses and static magnetic field pulses
    b. static magnetic field pulses and magnetic field gradient pulses
    c. magnetic field gradient pulses and RF pulses
    d. only RF pulses

11. How many general categories of pulse sequences are employed in MRI?

    a. 1   c. 3
    b. 2   d. 4

12. A spin echo pulse sequence consists of the following train of RF pulses:

    a. 90^0. . .90^0. . .90^0. . .
    b. 90^0. . .180^0. . .90^0. . .180^0. . .
    c. 180^0. . .90^0. . .180^0. . .90^0. . .
    d. 180^0. . .180^0. . .180^0. . .

13. The time to echo (TE) is the time between the:

    a. 90^0 RF pulse and the 180^0 RF pulse
    b. 90^0 RF pulse and the spin echo
    c. 180^0 RF pulse and the spin echo
    d. 180^0 RF pulse and the next 90^0 RF pulse

14. In a double echo, spin echo pulse sequence, TE for the second echo is the time from the 90^0 RF pulse to the:

    a. first 180^0 RF pulse
    b. second 180^0 RF pulse
    c. first spin echo
    d. second spin echo

15. The inversion recovery pulse sequence consists of a train of:

    a. 90^0. . .90^0. . .90^0. . .
    b. 90^0. . .180^0. . .180^0. . .
    c. 90^0. . .180^0. . .90^0. . .180^0. . .
    d. 180^0. . .90^0. . .180^0. . .90^0. . .

16. The inversion delay time (TI) is the time between:

    a. the 90^0 and the 180^0 RF pulse
    b. the 180^0 and the 90^0 RF pulse
    c. the 90^0 and the spin echo
    d. the 180^0 and the spin echo

17. The repetition time (TR) is the time:

    a. between the first RF signal and the spin echo
    b. between the first RF signal and the FID
    c. of slice acquisition
    d. from the start of one sequence to the next similar sequence

18. Which of the following pulse sequences involves all three—TR, TE and TI?

    a. saturation recovery
    b. inversion recovery
    c. spin echo
    d. gradient echo

19. In a double spin echo imaging sequence, which of the following signals would be most intense?

    a. the FID
    b. the first spin echo
    c. the second spin echo
    d. they are all the same

20. The figure below represents what type of pulse sequence?

    a. partial saturation   c. gradient echo
    b. spin echo   d. inversion recovery

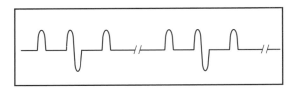

21. The figure below represents what type of pulse sequence?

    a. partial saturation   c. gradient echo
    b. spin echo   d. inversion recovery

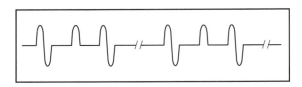

❑ QUESTIONS TO PONDER

22. How can TR/TE be compared to the radiographic parameters kVp and mAs?

23. What parameters can the operator adjust to obtain either a more T1W or T2W image?

24. In general, what is the value of a T2-weighted CSE image?

25. What is the relationship between short TR and saturation?

26. How does scan time vary when the number of phase encoding steps is changed?

Worksheet | 34

FID/SE/GE

1. Of the available net magnetization, the only one that can be observed during an MR imaging process is:

   a. M_b c. M_{xy}
   b. M_0 d. M_z

2. As M_{xy} relaxes to zero:
   (1) signal intensity decreases
   (2) signal intensity increases
   (3) an FID is produced
   (4) nothing happens

   a. 1, 2, and 3   c. 2 and 4
   b. 1 and 3   d. all are correct

3. The free induction decay is characterized as:
   (1) a constant signal for a short time
   (2) a signal decreasing in intensity
   (3) a signal increasing in intensity
   (4) a signal oscillating at the Larmor frequency

   a. 1, 2, and 3   c. 2 and 4
   b. 1 and 3   d. 4

4. At any point in time the intensity of the MR signal is proportional to the size of:

   a. M_b c. M_{xy}
   b. M_0 d. M_z

5. The primary MR signal is called a:

   a. relaxation signal
   b. free induction decay
   c. spin echo
   d. gradient-refocussed echo

6. Following the return of net magnetization to equilibrium, the MR signal:
   (1) is constant
   (2) is decreasing
   (3) oscillates at the Larmor frequency
   (4) is zero

   a. 1, 2, and 3   c. 2 and 4
   b. 1 and 3   d. 4

7. As M_z relaxes to equilibrium:

   a. signal intensity decreases
   b. signal intensity increases
   c. an FID is produced
   d. nothing happens

8. At equilibrium, if a 90^0 RF pulse is employed, which of the following MR signals will be produced?

   a. relaxation signal
   b. free induction decay
   c. spin echo
   d. gradient-refocussed echo

9. A free induction decay will be produced by a _____ RF pulse followed by a _____ RF pulse.

   a. 90^0, 90^0 c. 180^0, 180^0
   b. 90^0, 180^0 d. 180^0, 90^0

10. Control of TE is exercised by control of:

    a. the 90^0 RF pulse
    b. the 180^0 RF pulse
    c. the T1 relaxation time
    d. the T2 relaxation time

11. The MR signal called a spin echo is sometimes referred to as a:

    a. relaxation echo
    b. ghost echo
    c. free-induction decay
    d. gradient-refocussed echo

12. A spin echo appears:

    a. immediately after a 90^0 RF pulse
    b. immediately after a 180^0 RF pulse
    c. sometime following a 90^0 RF pulse
    d. sometime following a 180^0 RF pulse

13. Using the inversion recovery pulse sequence, MR images are constructed from:

a. free-induction decays
b. spin echoes
c. gradient-refocussed echoes
d. inversion echoes

14. A spin echo is a _____ MR signal.

a. primary
b. secondary
c. constant
d. off resonance

15. The time to echo (TE) is:
(1) the time between 90^0 and 180^0 RF pulses
(2) one half the time of the 90^0 RF pulse to the spin echo
(3) the time from the 180^0 RF pulse to the spin echo
(4) the time from the 90^0 RF pulse to the spin echo

a. 1, 2, and 3
b. 1 and 3
c. 2 and 4
d. 4

16 A spin echo is created when a _____ RF pulse is followed by a _____ RF pulse.

a. 90^0, 90^0
b. 90^0, 180^0
c. 180^0, 180^0
d. 180^0, 90^0

17. The time to echo (TE) is determined by the:

a. time of the 90^0 RF pulse
b. time of the 180^0 RF pulse
c. repetition time
d. time between the 90^0 and 180^0 RF pulses

18. Gradient echoes are required when _____ is required.
(1) best spatial resolution
(2) best contrast resolution
(3) low noise
(4) short exam time

a. 1, 2, and 3
b. 1 and 3
c. 2 and 4
d. 4

19. The principle characteristic of acquiring a gradient echo is:

a. the use of a 90^0 RF pulse
b. the use of an alpha RF pulse
c. the change in T1 relaxation time
d. the change in T2 relaxation time

20. Which of the drawings in the following figure symbolizes a varying phase encoding gradient pulse?

a. A
b. B
c. C
d. D

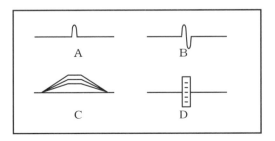

21. Match the following flip angles with the appropriate vector diagram in the figure below.

a. 0^0 RF _____
b. 10^0 RF _____
c. 30^0 RF _____
d. 180^0 RF _____

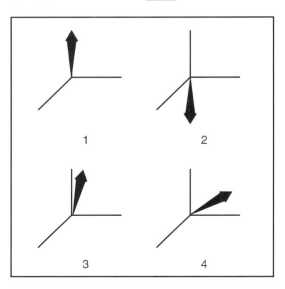

☐ QUESTIONS TO PONDER

22. Why is vascular lumen patency and hemorrhage visualized on MRI?

23. What are characteristics of the Inversion Recovery (IR) pulse sequence?

24. What two technical parameters will the MRI operator adjust to optimize image contrast?

25. Can time of flight (TOF) and phase contrast (PC) be imaged in 2D and 3D?

26. How is magnetic field inhomogeneity reflected in T2* and a T2 image?

PART TWO: DATA MANIPULATION

Worksheet | 35

The Fourier Transform

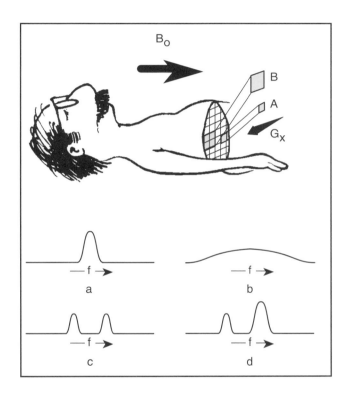

1. In MRI the role of the Fourier transform is to:

    a. precisely shape the magnetic field
    b. change the MR signal into an image
    c. separate T1 from T2
    d. measure the frequency bandwidth of the MR signal

2. The source function in MRI is a plot of:

    a. intensity vs time   c. intensity vs length
    b. intensity vs 1/time d. intensity vs 1/length

3. The Fourier transformation of a spin echo results in information in the:

    a. time domain   c. length domain
    b. frequency domain   d. volume domain

4. In the spatial frequency domain, sharp-edged objects:

    a. contain high frequencies
    b. approach a single frequency
    c. contain a narrow range of frequencies
    d. are independent of frequency

5. The two objects shown in the figure to the left are of the same tissue and in a magnetic field gradient. Object B is larger than object A. Which of the spatial frequency representations is most accurate?

6. The Fourier transformation of a symmetric spin echo will result in:

    a. a real part equal to zero
    b. an imaginary part equal to zero
    c. a function in the time domain
    d. a source function

7. Optimum sampling of an MR signal requires that a value be determined:

    a. at least once a cycle
    b. at least twice a cycle
    c. at least three times a cycle
    d. more than four times a cycle

8. When a square wave function is Fourier transformed (refer to the following figure), the result is:

   a. A
   b. B
   c. C
   d. D

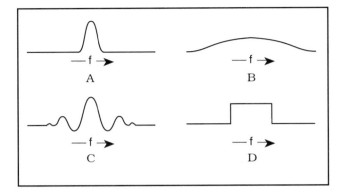

9. The result of a Fourier transform in MRI is called a (an):

   a. source function
   b. object function
   c. image function
   d. transform function

10. When a representation in the time domain is transformed into the frequency domain, units are transformed from _____ to _____.

    a. seconds, hertz
    b. hertz, seconds
    c. millimeters, millimeters^{-1}
    d. millimeters^{-1}, millimeters

11. In MRI smooth objects are represented by:

    a. zero frequency
    b. low frequencies
    c. high frequencies
    d. a wide range of frequencies

12. Slice selection during MR imaging requires a magnetic field gradient and:

    a. a shaped RF pulse
    b. a single frequency RF pulse
    c. an inverse RF pulse
    d. a flat RF pulse

13. MR signals received from moving tissue, e.g., flowing blood:

    a. contain non-zero imaginary parts when Fourier transformed
    b. contain zero real parts when Fourier transformed
    c. result in symmetric signals
    d. produce even functions

14. In MRI, sampling is the process of:

    a. detecting the MR signal
    b. transforming the MR signal
    c. changing the MR signal from a source function to a transformed function
    d. changing the MR signal from continuous to discrete

15. Aliasing in MR imaging results in the appearance of:

    a. a herringbone pattern
    b. wraparound objects
    c. distortion in the center of the image
    d. distortion at the periphery of the image

16. If the symbol FT stands for Fourier transform, the symbol FT^{-1} stands for:

    a. negative Fourier transform
    b. imaginary Fourier transform
    c. real Fourier transform
    d. inverse Fourier transform

17. The Fourier transformation of an MRI signal results in a function that is a plot of:

    a. intensity vs time
    b. intensity vs 1/time
    c. intensity vs length
    d. intensity vs 1/length

18. When an MR signal is Fourier transformed into the frequency domain, the result is

    a. slice selection
    b. an NMR spectrum
    c. a volume element
    d. a gradient echo

19. To truncate an MR signal is to:

    a. Fourier transform that signal
    b. intensify the signal artificially
    c. expand the range of frequencies in the signal
    d. chop off the frequency range abruptly

20. The shape of the RF pulse used for slice selection is determined with the use of a:

    a. Fourier transform
    b. inverse Fourier transform
    c. gradient pulse
    d. inverse gradient pulse

21. The process of sampling is performed by:

    a. an analog to digital converter (ADC)
    b. a free-induction decay (FID)
    c. a Fourier transform (FT)
    d. the inverse Fourier transform (FT^{-1})

22. When a spin echo is Fourier transformed, the result appears as (refer to the following figure):

a. A   c. C
b. B   d. D

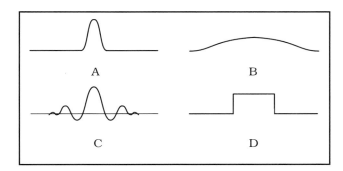

23. A spin echo is a plot of:

a. intensity vs time   c. intensity vs length
b. intensity vs 1/time d. intensity vs 1/length

24. When a spin echo is Fourier transformed, the result is a representation in:
(1) Fourier space
(2) frequency space
(3) spatial frequency
(4) source domain

a. 1, 2, and 3   c. 2 and 4
b. 1 and 3   d. all are correct

25. If a spin echo is truncated and Fourier transformed, the result appears as (refer to the following figure):

a. A   c. C
b. B   d. D

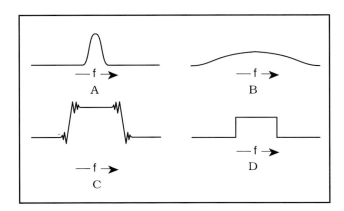

26. The Fourier transformation of a function from the time domain to the frequency domain has two components that are called:

a. A and B   c. plus and minus
b. X and Y   d. real and imaginary

27. The abbreviation FFT stands for:

a. first Fourier transform
b. final Fourier transform
c. fast Fourier transform
d. fudged Fourier transform

28. The mathematical form of any Fourier transform contains:

a. a's and b's
b. bits and bytes
c. pluses and minuses
d. sines and cosines

29. When a spin echo is Fourier transformed, the result is:

a. an FID   c. an NMR spectrum
b. a gradient echo d. a RF pulse

30. The Fourier transformation of an MR signal results in:
(1) an NMR spectrum
(2) the source domain
(3) a spatial frequency plot
(4) an image

a. 1, 2, and 3   c. 2 and 4
b. 1 and 3   d. 4

31. The range of frequencies observed in the Fourier transformation of an MR signal from a single tissue is due to:

a. discontinuities within that tissue
b. magnetic field gradients
c. the type of RF pulse sequence
d. the magnetic shim field

32. The Fourier transformation of an even time domain function results in a spatial frequency function:
(1) with an imaginary part that is zero
(2) with all non-zero information in the imaginary part
(3) that is symmetric about the vertical axis
(4) containing all high frequencies

a. 1, 2, and 3   c. 2 and 4
b. 1 and 3   d. 4

33. The Fourier transform of a discrete function, e.g., a sampled MRI signal, is a:

   a. discrete function
   b. continuous function
   c. single frequency
   d. single dimension

34. When applying a Fourier transform, the MRI signal is identified as the:

   a. source function   c. image function
   b. object function   d. transform function

35. When a spin echo is Fourier transformed, the result has dimensions of:

   a. intensity vs time   c. intensity vs length
   b. intensity vs 1/time   d. intensity vs 1/length

36. Which of the drawings in the following figure best represents the Fourier transformation of a frequency spectrum?

   a. A   c. C
   b. B   d. D

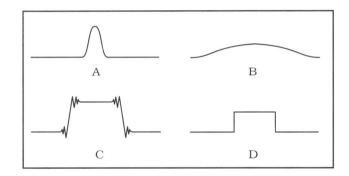

37. In a uniform magnetic field the two objects shown in the figure below would result in a spatial frequency representation shown by which diagram?

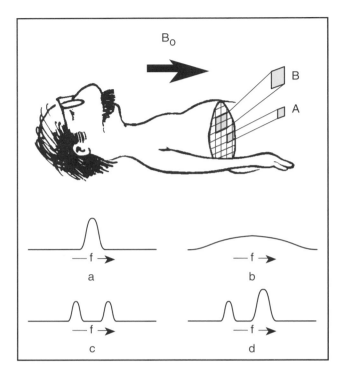

38. Which of the graphs in the following figure is an even function?

   a. A   c. C
   b. B   d. D

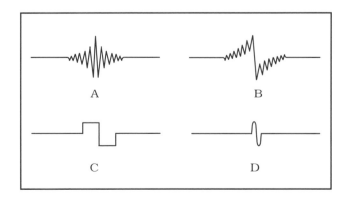

39. If the sampling rate of an MR signal is insufficient, the result is an artifact called:

  a. truncation
  b. Gibbs' phenomena
  c. magnetic susceptibility
  d. aliasing

40. When a spin echo is Fourier transformed, the answer is in:

  a. Fourier space   c. Fourier frequency
  b. Fourier time   d. Fourier length

41. As an MR signal becomes more narrow in time, it:

  a. contains a wider range of frequencies
  b. approaches a single frequency emission
  c. has greater intensity
  d. is more likely to generate artifacts

42. The spatial frequency representation of two objects of the same material and the same size, as in the figure below (no magnetic field gradient), should appear as:

43. Which of the functions in the following figure will have a Fourier transform function with an imaginary part equal to zero?

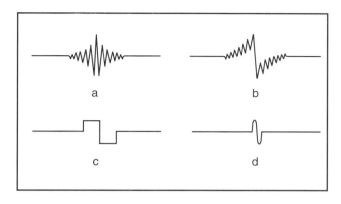

□ **QUESTIONS TO PONDER**

44. Why is more data sampling desirable?

45. Can a Fourier transformation be done without a computer?

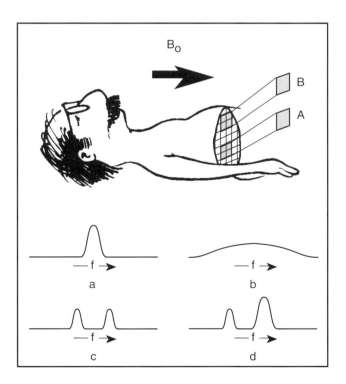

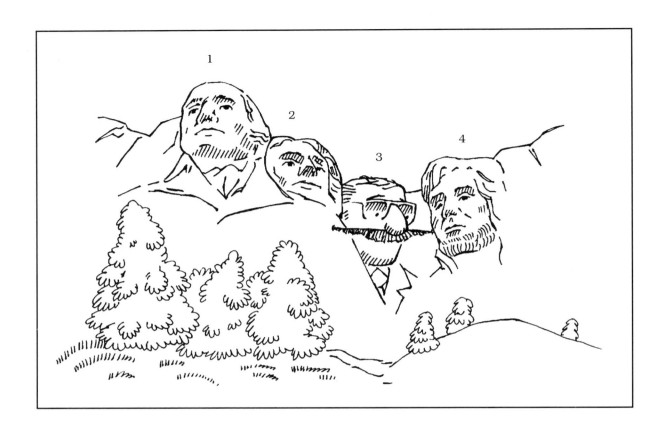

Match the face to the appropriate description.

a. Led us out of the Civil War   ____
b. Our first president   ____
c. Author of the Declaration of
    Independence   ____
d. Golf handicap = 23   ____

Worksheet | 36

Spatial Frequency

1. The term spatial frequency domain is borrowed from:

   a. physics
   b. biology
   c. computer science
   d. electrical engineering

2. When one mentions a frequency measured in megahertz, one is talking about:

   a. spatial frequency
   b. temporal frequency
   c. energy frequency
   d. volume frequency

3. Match the following:
   (1) X,Y
   (2) hertz
   (3) cycles per millimeter
   (4) X, α

   a. temporal frequency _____
   b. spatial frequency _____
   c. polar coordinates _____
   d. Cartesian coordinates _____

4. The mathematical tool used to analyze the frequency content of an object is the:

   a. induction transform
   b. Fourier transform
   c. imaginary number rule
   d. Cartesian number rule

5. For a high resolution image _____ must be measured.

   a. high spin densities
   c. high spatial frequencies
   b. low spin densities
   d. low spatial frequencies

6. Noise in an image is generally more apparent when _____ are present.

   a. high spatial frequencies
   b. low spatial frequencies
   c. short relaxation times
   d. long relaxation times

7. Adjacent pixels having great difference in brightness represent:

   a. low spatial frequency
   b. high spatial frequency
   c. low temporal frequency
   d. high temporal frequency

8. The spatial frequency domain of an MR image is sampled in a:

   a. single line
   b. rectangular raster
   c. circular projectory
   d. elliptical projectory

9. The first method employed to reconstruct data for an MR image was:

   a. two-dimensional Fourier transformation
   b. three-dimensional Fourier transformation
   c. filtered back projection
   d. forward, reverse transformation

10. The middle region of the spatial frequency domain is that which determines:

    a. spatial resolution
    b. contrast resolution
    c. spin density information
    d. relaxation time data

11. The term k-space is borrowed from:

    a. physics
    b. biology
    c. computer science
    d. electrical engineering

12. Complex numbers used in MRI have two parts identified as:

    a. north, south   c. real, imaginary
    b. east, west   d. X, Y

13. The different positions of the net magnetization vector along a row of voxels represents:

    a. spatial frequency
    b. temporal frequency
    c. spin density
    d. relaxation time

14. The raw data of an MRI signal contains the _____ of the spatial frequencies.

    a. x and y coordinates
    b. angle and intensity
    c. intensity and frequency
    d. magnitude and phase

15. Field of view (FOV) relates to the:

    a. diameter of the patient aperture of the imager
    b. maximum diameter of the patient
    c. diameter of the area that is reconstructed
    d. the diameter of a pixel

16. In general, when one samples the data of the spatial frequency domain with emphasis on the higher spatial frequencies:

    a. the examination will take longer
    b. the field of view will be larger
    c. the signal-to-noise ratio will be less
    d. the spatial resolution will be less

17. Two pixels having different brightness and positioned far apart represent:

    a. low spatial frequency
    b. high spatial frequency
    c. low temporal frequency
    d. high temporal frequency

18. The trajectory in k-space refers to:

    a. each X and Y point
    b. each angle and distance
    c. the method of sampling the spatial frequency domain
    d. the method of sampling the temporal frequency domain

19. The spatial frequency domain can also be sampled by:
    (1) spiral scanning
    (2) square spiral scanning
    (3) interleaved spiral scanning
    (4) alternate direction line scanning

    a. 1, 2, and 3   c. 2 and 4
    b. 1 and 3   d. all are correct

20. Frequency is measured in units of:

    a. joules   c. hertz
    b. meters   d. electron volts

21. Using polar coordinates, a point is represented by:

    a. an X value and a Y value
    b. a real value and an imaginary value
    c. the distance from the origin and angle from the X axis
    d. the angle from the x axis and angle from the Y axis

22. An entire object can be viewed as the weighted sum of:

    a. spatial frequencies
    b. temporal frequencies
    c. spin density
    d. relaxation times

23. The spatial frequency information collected as MRI signals is converted to an image by:

    a. reconstruction projection techniques
    b. induction transformation techniques
    c. spin density transformation
    d. Fourier transformation

24. The signal-to-noise ratio (SNR) determines:

    a. how much of the patient will be imaged
    b. how grainy the image will appear
    c. the spatial frequency range of the image
    d. the relationship of transverse relaxation to longitudinal relaxation

25. Noise in an MR image is generally related to what property of the spatial frequency domain?

    a. number of lines
    b. length of lines
    c. the higher spatial frequencies
    d. the lower spatial frequencies

26. Contrast in an MR image is generally determined by:

    a. low spatial frequencies
    b. high spatial frequencies
    c. low temporal frequencies
    d. high temporal frequencies

27. Measuring the spatial frequency domain of an object will result in:

    a. an image of the object
    b. the noise in the object
    c. the size of the object
    d. the temporal resolution of the object

28. Sampling the spatial frequency domain is controlled by:

    a. the B_0 magnetic field
    b. magnetic field gradients
    c. the transmitted RF signal
    d. the received RF signal

29. In conventional MR imaging, the spatial frequency domain is scanned:

    a. from top to bottom
    b. from bottom to top
    c. from the middle out
    d. from the outer edges in

30. One hertz is equal to one:

    a. cycle per centimeter
    b. cycle per meter
    c. cycle per second
    d. cycle per eV

31. When specifying frequency in hertz, one cycle equals:

    a. one second   c. 180^0
    b. one minute   d. 360^0

32. One obtains the appearance of an object from the spatial frequencies in that object by using:

    a. spin density weights
    b. relaxation time weights
    c. induction transformation
    d. Fourier transformation

33. Improving spatial resolution in an image requires that _____ be sampled.

    a. higher spin densities
    b. lower spin densities
    c. higher spatial frequencies
    d. lower spatial frequencies

34. Most images have more signal at:
    (1) high spin density
    (2) low spin density
    (3) low spatial frequencies
    (4) high spatial frequencies

    a. 1, 2, and 3   c. 2 and 4
    b. 1 and 3   d. 4

35. When reconstructing an MR image, there is always a trade-off between:
    (1) spatial resolution and temporal resolution
    (2) transverse and longitudinal relaxation times
    (3) spatial frequencies sampled and noise
    (4) noise and spatial resolution

    a. 1, 2, and 3   c. 2 and 4
    b. 1 and 3   d. 4

36. In two-dimensional Fourier transform (2DFT) imaging, the spatial frequency domain is measured:

    a. in a circular fashion
    b. in an elliptical fashion
    c. every line from left to right
    d. every line, but alternating direction

37. The term "segmented k-space" refers to sampling:

    a. all of the spatial frequency domain
    b. the top half of the spatial frequency domain
    c. the bottom half of the spatial frequency domain
    d. only a portion of the spatial frequency domain

38. The figure below is usually referred to as:
    (1) a longitudinal relaxation map
    (2) the spatial frequency domain
    (3) a transverse relaxation map
    (4) k-space

    a. 1, 2, and 3   c. 2 and 4
    b. 1 and 3   d. all are correct

39. Which letter in the figure below identifies the k_y axis?

    a. A   c. C
    b. B   d. D

40. Which letter in the figure below relates to strong phase encoding gradients?

    a. A   c. C
    b. B   d. D

41. Which letter in the following figure relates to course, high contrast features in an image?

    a. A   c. C
    b. B   d. D

☐ **QUESTIONS TO PONDER**

42. What two properties of an MR signal are analyzed in order to obtain its exact "spatial address"?

43. What happens to image contrast when a second pulse sequence is applied before complete relaxation?

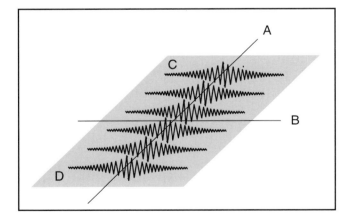

Worksheet | 37 |

Spin Echo Techniques

1. Match the following physiologic motions with their appropriate time:
   (1) 1 ms; (2) 200 ms; (3) 2 s; (4) 8 s

   a. swallowing _____
   b. peristalsis _____
   c. nervous action potential _____
   d. blinking _____

2. When the Y gradient of a superconducting magnet is identified as the slice select gradient, the image plane is:

   a. transverse   c. coronal
   b. sagittal   d. oblique

3. When constructing an image, the matrix size is equal to the number of different:

   a. RF pulses transmitted into the patient
   b. slice select gradients applied
   c. phase-encoding gradients applied
   d. frequency-encoding gradients applied

4. Lines of the spatial frequency domain acquired with weak phase encoding gradients principally contribute information about:
   (1) large smooth objects
   (2) small sharp objects
   (3) contrast resolution
   (4) spatial resolution

   a. 1, 2, and 3   c. 2 and 4
   b. 1 and 3   d. 4 only is correct

5. For the inversion recovery pulse sequence the MR signal detected can be:
   (1) an FID
   (2) a gradient echo
   (3) a planar echo
   (4) a spin echo

   a. 1, 2, and 3   c. 2 and 4
   b. 1 and 3   d. 4

6. STIR sequences can be designed to suppress the signal from fat because fat has a:

   a. long TR   c. short T1
   b. long TE   d. short T2

7. In order to employ artifact free imaging, _____ is required.

   a. a sufficiently long TR
   b. at least 128 signal acquisitions
   c. symmetry in the spatial frequency domain
   d. a long inversion time

8. In FSE the zero order spin echo is that which follows the:

   a. first 180^0 RF pulse
   b. last 180^0 RF pulse
   c. weakest phase-encoding gradient pulse
   d. strongest phase-encoding gradient pulse

9. Temporal resolution is a term applied to:

   a. the accurate determination of temperature
   b. time-related events
   c. temporary resolution
   d. tables of temperature

10. When the X magnetic field gradient of a superconducting magnet is applied as the slice select gradient, the image plane is:

    a. transverse   c. coronal
    b. sagittal   d. oblique

11. To construct a 128 x 128 image matrix, 128 different values of _____ must be applied.

    a. RF pulses
    b. slice select gradients
    c. phase-encoding gradients
    d. frequency-encoding gradients

12. Lines of the spatial frequency domain obtained with strong phase encoding gradients are located:

   a. on the periphery of the spatial frequency domain
   b. in the center of the spatial frequency domain
   c. interleaved throughout the spatial frequency domain
   d. just outside the spatial frequency domain

13. The inversion recovery pulse sequence is identified as

   a. $90^0...90^0...90^0...$
   b. $90^0...180^0...90^0...180^0...$
   c. $180^0...90^0...180^0...90^0...$
   d. $180^0...180^0...180^0...$

14. The FLAIR pulse sequence is:
   (1) a stir sequence with a shorter TI
   (2) a stir sequence with a longer TI
   (3) Find Late Activity In Recovery
   (4) Fluid Attenuated Inversion Recovery

   a. 1, 2, and 3   c. 2 and 4
   b. 1 and 3   d. 4

15. The CPMG pulse sequence is applied in:

   a. spin echo imaging
   b. gradient echo imaging
   c. MR angiography
   d. echo planar imaging

16. The phase-encoding gradient is energized:

   a. during signal detection
   b. at the time of the RF pulse
   c. at the beginning of the FID
   d. in the middle of the frequency encoding

17. CSE is short for _____ pulse sequence.

   a. conventional spin echo
   b. contemporary spin echo
   c. classical spin echo
   d. crossed spin echo

18. Weak phase-encoding gradients are associated with:

   a. low spatial frequencies
   b. high spatial frequencies
   c. a single spatial frequency
   d. random spatial frequencies

19. The inversion recovery pulse sequence is used for:

   a. faster imaging time
   b. better T1 contrast
   c. better T2 contrast
   d. better spin density contrast

20. The following pulse sequences use inversion recovery technique:
   (1) IRM
   (2) ABSIR
   (3) STIR
   (4) FLAIR

   a. 1, 2, and 3   c. 2 and 4
   b. 1 and 3   d. all are correct

21. The fast spin echo pulse sequence (FSE) can be described as:

   a. $90^0...90^0...90^0...$
   b. $90^0...180^0...180^0...180^0...$
   c. $180^0...180^0...180^0...180^0...$
   d. $180^0...90^0...90^0...90^0...$

22. The term pulse sequence as applied in MRI refers to:
   (1) the timing of RF pulses
   (2) detecting the MR signal
   (3) applying magnetic field gradients
   (4) identification of image plane

   a. 1, 2, and 3   c. 2 and 4
   b. 1 and 3   d. all are correct

23. The read gradient is also known as the:

   a. slice select gradient
   b. frequency-encoding gradient
   c. phase-encoding gradient
   d. RF-encoding gradient

24. The principle difference between conventional spin echo (CSE) and fast spin echo (FSE) is:

   a. a shorter TR
   b. a shorter TE
   c. multiple spin echoes within one TR
   d. multiple spin echoes within one TI

25. The spatial frequency domain, k-space, in CSE is filled:

   a. in sequential order
   b. in an interleaved fashion
   c. segmentally
   d. randomly

26. The contrast rendition of FSE imaging is best related to:

a. T1 weighted
b. T1* weighted
c. T2 weighted
d. T2* weighted

27. Strong phase encoding gradients are associated with:

a. low spatial frequencies
b. high spatial frequencies
c. a single spatial frequency
d. random spatial frequencies

28. Which of the TEs shown in the following figure is the effective echo time?

a. TE1
b. TE2
c. TE3
d. TE4

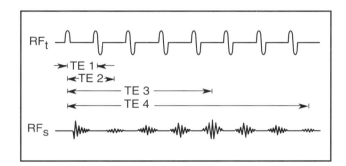

29. Inversion recovery imaging allows for the:

a. amplification of signal from a given tissue
b. nulling of a signal from a given tissue
c. speeding examination time
d. speeding patient throughput

30. Partial Fourier imaging is possible because of:

a. long repetition times
b. long echo times
c. high magnetic field strengths
d. Hermitian symmetry

31. The slice select gradient is always applied:

a. during signal detection
b. with the phase-encoding gradient
c. with the frequency-encoding gradient
d. at the time of the RF pulse

32. During the time that the frequency encoding gradient is energized:

a. RF is transmitted into the patient
b. an MR signal is received from the patient
c. the patient will be relaxed
d. the patient will be at equilibrium

33. Lines of the spatial frequency domain acquired with weak phase encoding gradients are:

a. on the periphery of the spatial frequency domain
b. in the middle of the spatial frequency domain
c. interleaved throughout the spatial frequency domain
d. randomly distributed throughout the spatial frequency domain

34. Image artifacts occur if:
(1) the subject changes position to one TR interval to the next
(2) the TR is shorter than arrhythmic motion
(3) there is motion while the read gradient is on
(4) each spin echo is symmetric

a. 1, 2, and 3
b. 1 and 3
c. 2 and 4
d. all are correct

35. STIR stands for:

a. safe time in recovery
b. sequence time in relaxation
c. soft tune inversion RF
d. short time inversion recovery

36. Half Fourier imaging uses:

(1) the top half of the spatial frequency domain
(2) the bottom half of the spatial frequency domain
(3) the left side of the spatial frequency domain
(4) the right side of the spatial frequency domain

a. 1, 2, and 3
b. 1 and 3
c. 2 and 4
d. all are correct

37. The spin echo train measured in FSE experiences _____ from one echo to the next.

a. T1 relaxation
b. T2 relaxation
c. spin density modification
d. non symmetry effects

38. Which pulse sequence can be used for contrast reversal?

39. How is the scan time affected by a double spin echo pulse sequence compared to a single spin echo pulse sequence?

40. Why are flow-related spins more sensitive than stationary spins in spin echo imaging?

41. What are characteristics of fast spin echo (FSE) imaging?

42. Where would one likely use longer repetion times (TR)?

Gradient Echo Techniques

1. Gradient echo imaging is characterized by:

   a. a single 90(RF pulse
   b. a refocussing magnetic field gradient
   c. shorter T1 relaxation times
   d. shorter T2 relaxation times

2. Gradient echoes are also known as:
   (1) gradient-transformed echoes
   (2) gradient-refocussed echoes
   (3) reformatted echoes
   (4) gradient-recalled echoes

   a. 1, 2, and 3   c. 2 and 4
   b. 1 and 3   d. 4

3. Unlike spin echoes, gradient echoes are influenced by:

   a. random motions of molecules
   b. irreversible magnetic field inhomogeneities
   c. reversible magnetic field inhomogeneities
   d. T1 relaxation influences

4. Which of the following are gradient echo pulse sequences?
   (1) gradient-recalled acquisition at steady state
   (2) fast imaging with steady state precession
   (3) fast low angle shot
   (4) rapid acquired relaxation enhanced technique

   a. 1, 2, and 3   c. 2 and 4
   b. 1 and 3   d. 4

5. When a sequence of pulses reduces longitudinal relaxation by the same amount that is recovered between pulses, the result is:
   (1) T1 amplification
   (2) an equilibrium state
   (3) T2 amplification
   (4) a steady state

   a. 1, 2, and 3   c. 2 and 4
   b. 1 and 3   d. all are correct

6. Following a 30^0 flip angle, transverse magnetization has a value of:

   a. 1%   c. 50%
   b. 58%   d. 87%

7. The gradient echo pulse sequence can be identified as:

   a. alpha . . .alpha . . .alpha . . .alpha
   b. 90^0. . .90^0. . .90^0. . .
   c. 90^0. . .180^0. . .90^0. . .180^0
   d. 180^0. . .90^0. . .180^0. . .90^0

8. When compared with T2, T2*:

   a. is always shorter   c. will depend on T1
   b. is always longer   d. will depend on T1*

9. T2* is shorter than T2 principally because of:

   a. differences in T1
   b. differences in T2
   c. the influence of reversible magnetic field inhomogeneities
   d. the influence of irreversible magnetic field inhomogeneities

10. Stimulated echoes occur as a consequence of:

    a. T2 relaxation
    b. T2* relaxation
    c. equilibrium magnetization
    d. magnetization steady state

11. Long repetition times (TR) result in:

    a. accelerated T1 relaxation
    b. accelerated T2 relaxation
    c. longitudinal magnetization that is close to equilibrium
    d. transverse magnetization that is close to equilibrium

12. At what flip angle does the transverse magnetization equal 0.5 M_0?

    a. 15°   c. 60°
    b. 30°   d. 75°

13. An alpha pulse is:

    a. an RF pulse less than 90°
    b. an RF pulse between 90° and 180°
    c. a pulsed magnetic field gradient
    d. a pulsed signal reception

14. Which of the following pulse sequences does not use a 180° RF pulse?
    (1) partial saturation
    (2) echo planar
    (3) spin echo
    (4) gradient echo

    a. 1, 2, and 3   c. 2 and 4
    b. 1 and 3   d. 4 only is correct

15. A magnetic field gradient designed to inhibit the formation of a stimulated echo is called:

    a. a spoiler   c. a stimulator
    b. a steady state d. a truncation

16. With very low flip angle excitations:

    a. accelerated T1 relaxation occurs
    b. accelerated T2 relaxation occurs
    c. longitudinal magnetization is close to equilibrium
    d. transverse magnetization is close to equilibrium

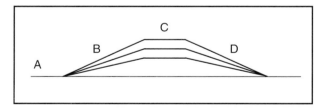

17. Which letter in the above figure relates to spins out of phase (phase incoherence)?

    a. A   c. C
    b. B   d. D

18. Which letter in the above figure relates to spins rephasing?

    a. A   c. C
    b. B   d. D

19. Which letter in the preceding figure relates to spins in phase (phase coherence)?

    a. A   c. C
    b. B   d. D

20. Irreversible magnetic field homogeneities include:
    (1) RF-induced fields
    (2) B_0 magnetic field imperfections
    (3) transient magnetic effects
    (4) magnetic susceptibility differences

    a. 1, 2, and 3   c. 2 and 4
    b. 1 and 3   d. 4

21. When compared with a spin echo, a gradient echo:

    a. is less intense
    b. takes a longer time
    c. is more T2 dependent
    d. is more T1 dependent

22. When stimulated echoes are suppressed, images are usually:

    a. of high contrast
    b. of high spatial resolution
    c. strongly T1 weighted
    d. strongly T2 weighted

23. Following an alpha RF pulse, the magnetization that produces an MR signal is that:

    a. projected onto the +Z axis
    b. projected onto the -Z axis
    c. projected onto the XY plane
    d. which is T1 relaxed

❏ QUESTIONS TO PONDER

24. What RF pulse sequence produces a rapid series of different spin echos?

25. What is the relationship between saturated vs. unsaturated spins in vascular image contrast?

26. In general, where is a presaturation RF pulse applied?

27. How does the geometry of the blood vessel affect blood flow velocity?

28. What image weighting is generally created by fast scanning techniques?

Worksheet | 39

Purpose of Pulse Sequences

1. A pulse sequence diagram should contain the following lines of data:
   (1) MRI signal acquired
   (2) slice selection gradient
   (3) transmitted RF pulse
   (4) phase-encoding magnetic field gradient

   a. 1, 2, and 3   c. 2 and 4
   b. 1 and 3   d. all are correct

2. Unlike x-ray imaging, the contrast rendition in MRI is:

   a. always the same   c. less
   b. reversable   d. random

3. The character of a pixel element refers to its:

   a. size   c. location
   b. brightness   d. depth

4. The brightness of a pixel in a CT image is determined by _____ while that for an MR image is determined by _____.

   a. time, space
   b. attenuation coefficient, matrix size
   c. attenuation coefficient, spin density
   d. relaxation time, spin density

5. For completeness, an MR pulse sequence diagram should contain at least _____ lines of information.

   a. one   c. five
   b. three   d. seven

6. The two principle timing patterns in a pulse sequence diagram are:

   a. temporal resolution and contrast resolution
   b. temporal resolution and spatial resolution
   c. RF pulses and exposure time
   d. RF pulses and magnetic field gradients

7. The two properties of any picture element are:

   a. size and depth
   b. depth and character
   c. character and position
   d. position and size

8. In an MR image a pixel emitting an intense MR signal would be rendered:

   a. black   c. light gray
   b. dark gray   d. bright

9. A pulse sequence is:

   a. a mathematical algorithm
   b. the result of a Fourier transformation
   c. a time line diagram of MR operation
   d. the name of a controlling subassembly of an MR imager

10. The contrast rendition of an MR image is principally determined by:

    a. the number of signal acquisitions
    b. the gray scale resolution of the computer
    c. RF pulse amplitude and timing
    d. magnetic field gradient amplitude and timing

11. Spatial localization of signals in an MR imager is identified by:

    a. collimation   c. signal enhancement
    b. filtration   d. signal encoding

12. The position of a pixel element deals with its:

    a. size   c. location
    b. brightness   d. depth

13. The principle control of spatial resolution in an MR imager is determined by:

    a. the number of signal acquisitions
    b. the gray scale resolution of the computer
    c. RF pulse amplitude and timing
    d. magnetic field gradient amplitude and timing

14. Regardless of the type of magnet the Z axis is always:

    a. horizontal   c. parallel with the B_0 field
    b. vertical   d. across the patient

15. For a superconducting magnet the Z axis is:
    (1) vertical
    (2) horizontal
    (3) across the patient
    (4) along B_0

    a. 1, 2, and 3   c. 2 and 4
    b. 1 and 3   d. 4

16. When all three pairs of magnetic field gradient coils are energized simultaneously, the result is a magnetic field gradient:
    (1) along one axis
    (2) circularly
    (3) in an orthogonal plane
    (4) in an oblique plane

    a. 1, 2, and 3   c. 2 and 4
    b. 1 and 3   d. 4

17. Which of the drawings in the figure below depicts the coordinate system for a superconducting magnet?

    a. A   c. C
    b. B   d. D

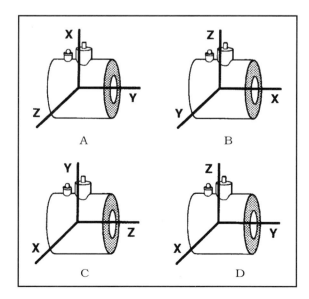

18. A B_0 magnetic field that is uniform throughout the imaging volume is said to be:

    a. intense   c. heterogeneous
    b. relaxed   d. homogeneous

19. When a single pair of magnetic field gradient coils is energized, a magnetic field gradient is produced:
    (1) along one axis
    (2) circularly
    (3) in an orthogonal plane
    (4) in an oblique plane

    a. 1, 2, and 3   c. 2 and 4
    b. 1 and 3   d. 4

20. Which of the drawings in the following figure corresponds to the coordinate system used for vector diagrams?

    a. A   c. C
    b. B   d. D

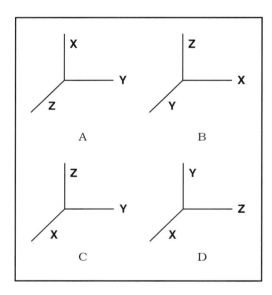

□ QUESTIONS TO PONDER

21. Why do proteins often appear brighter on MRI than water?

22. What does bipolar refer to in the gradient echo pulse sequence?

23. What happens if the TR is too long when performing MRA?

24. What are the two basic MRA pulse sequences?

25. What is the relationship between flip angle and signal-to-noise ratio (S/N)?

Function of Gradient Coils

1. Magnetic field gradients serve two principle purposes:

   a. slice selection and pixel location within a slice
   b. pixel location within a slice and pixel intensity
   c. pixel intensity and pixel character
   d. pixel character and slice selection

2. In order to excite spins in a given slice of tissue the RF pulse must:

   a. be turned on for a longer time
   b. be repeatedly energized
   c. match the Larmor frequency at B_o
   d. match the Larmor frequency at B_o plus G

3. Spins in a coronal slice in a superconducting imager are selectively excited when the _____ is (are) energized.

   a. X gradient   c. Z gradient
   b. Y gradient   d. X, Y, and Z gradients

4. The Q value of an RF pulse is expressed as the:

   a. square of the resonant frequency
   b. resonant frequency times the bandwidth
   c. resonant frequency divided by the bandwidth
   d. bandwidth divided by the resonant frequency

5. When two pixels exist in the same magnetic field and one is brighter than the other, it is probably brighter because of:

   a. higher spin density
   b. a stronger magnetic field gradient
   c. a more intense RF pulse
   d. the post-processing algorithm

6. The effect of the pulsed phase encoding gradient on the phase of spins along a column is:

   a. none
   b. to increase the phase perpendicular to the gradient
   c. to decrease the phase perpendicular to the gradient
   d. to impress a phase shift along the gradient

7. The frequency-encoding gradient is:

   a. pulsed at the same time as the phase-encoding gradient
   b. energized during RF excitation
   c. is energized during signal acquisition
   d. is energized following signal acquisition

8. The gyromagnetic ratio for hydrogen is equal to:

   a. 21 megahertz per tesla
   b. 42 megahertz per tesla
   c. 21 tesla per megahertz
   d. 42 tesla per megahertz

9. The selection of a slice of tissue for imaging requires:

   a. the absence of a magnetic field gradient
   b. a magnetic field gradient plus RF excitation
   c. RF excitation and MR signal acquisition
   d. magnetic field gradient and MR signal acquisition

10. Spins in an oblique slice in a superconducting imager are selectively excited when the _____ is (are) energized.

    a. X gradient   c. Z gradient
    b. Y gradient   d. X, Y, and Z gradients

11. Which of the following RF pulses should produce the thinnest slice in a 1 T imager?

    a. 42 ± 0.1 MHz   c. 63 ± 0.1 MHz
    b. 42 ± 0.5 MHz   d. 63 ± 0.5 MHz

12. For a transverse image acquired with a superconducting MR imager, columns are localized by _____ and rows by _____ .

    a. X axis frequency-encoding gradient, Y axis phase-encoding gradient
    b. X axis phase-encoding gradient, Y axis frequency-encoding gradient
    c. Y axis frequency-encoding gradient, X axis phase-encoding gradient
    d. Y axis phase-encoding gradient, X axis frequency-encoding gradient

13. The "spin warp" method refers to:

    a. the twisted change in frequency due to the RF pulse
    b. a twisted change in frequency during the gradient pulse
    c. a twisted change in frequency after the gradient pulse
    d. the phase shift impressed along the gradient

14. While the phase encoding gradient is pulsed with different amplitude for each signal acquisition, the frequency-encoding gradient is:
    (1) pulsed with different amplitude also
    (2) pulsed with the same amplitude
    (3) on during the RF pulse
    (4) on during signal acquisition

    a. 1, 2, and 3   c. 2 and 4
    b. 1 and 3   d. 4

15. A magnetic field gradient changes the homogeneity of the B_o magnetic field:

    a. linearly   c. exponentially
    b. circularly   d. normally

16. Pixel localization within a slice requires:

    a. the absence of a magnetic field gradient
    b. a magnetic field gradient plus RF excitation
    c. RF excitation and MR signal acquisition
    d. magnetic field gradient and MR signal acquisition

17. Slice thickness is determined by:
    (1) RF pulse flip angle
    (2) RF pulse bandwidth
    (3) magnetic field intensity
    (4) magnetic field gradient slope

    a. 1, 2, and 3   c. 2 and 4
    b. 1 and 3   d. 4

18. Which of the following Q values represents the thinnest slice?

    a. 10   c. 100
    b. 50   d. 500

19. Use of the rotating frame to describe precession in MRI:

    a. ignores the B_o field
    b. assumes a uniform B_o field
    c. requires a high Q RF pulse
    d. requires a broad bandpass RF pulse

20. The only row of voxels that contribute an MR signal during a given phase-encoding gradient is that row:

    a. with no twist
    b. with maximum twist
    c. with the same resonance frequency
    d. in the center of k-space

21. The frequency-encoding gradient allows measurement of the range of frequencies:

    a. along the phase encoding gradient direction
    b. along the frequency encoding direction
    c. in a slice
    d. in a volume

22. The application of a magnetic field gradient (G) causes spins along G to precess at:

    a. the same frequency
    b. a frequency proportional to B_o
    c. a frequency proportional to G
    d. a frequency proportional to gamma

23. Spins in a single transverse slice in a superconducting imager are selectively excited when the _____ is (are) energized.

    a. X gradient   c. Z gradient
    b. Y gradient   d. X, Y, and Z gradients

24. The slice of tissue imaged in MRI can be made thinner by increasing the:

   a. number of signal acquisitions
   b. RF pulse flip angle
   c. band pass of the RF pulse
   d. slope of the magnetic field gradient

25. Which of the following magnetic field gradients should result in the thinnest slice?

   a. 5 mT/m   c. 15 mT/s
   b. 10 mT/m   d. 20 mT/s

26. For vector diagram purposes, the MR technologist is said to be in a:
   (1) rotating frame
   (2) laboratory frame
   (3) circular frame
   (4) stationary frame

   a. 1, 2, and 3   c. 2 and 4
   b. 1 and 3   d. 4

27. In CSE, during each application of the frequency-encoding gradient:
   (1) an MR signal is acquired
   (2) an MR image is acquired
   (3) the horizontal spatial frequencies for one line are measured
   (4) the vertical spatial frequencies for one line are measured

   a. 1, 2, and 3   c. 2 and 4
   b. 1 and 3   d. 4

28. During phase encoding the only spatial frequency measured is the:

   a. maximum frequency in the signal
   b. minimum frequency in the signal
   c. frequency with maximum phase twist
   d. frequency with no phase twist

29. Spins in a row of voxels perpendicular to a magnetic field gradient (G) precess at:

   a. the same frequency
   b. frequencies proportional to Bo
   c. frequencies proportional to G
   d. different frequencies proportional to gamma

30. Spins in a sagittal slice in a superconducting imager are selectively excited when the _____ is (are) energized.

   a. X gradient   c. Z gradient
   b. Y gradient   d. X, Y, and Z gradients

31. The slice of tissue imaged in MRI can be made thinner by decreasing the:

   a. number of signal acquisitions
   b. RF pulse flip angle
   c. bandpass of the RF pulse
   d. slope of the magnetic field gradient

32. Magnetic field gradients are made more intense by:

   a. leaving them on longer
   b. pulsing the gradient coil excitation
   c. applying a higher voltage to the gradient coil
   d. running more current through the gradient coil

33. The effect of the pulsed phase encoding gradient on the frequency of a column of spins is:

   a. none
   b. to increase the frequency with increasing gradient
   c. to decrease the frequency with increasing gradient
   d. to reverse the frequency

34. During phase encoding to produce a phase shift, the sum of the phase shifts:

   a. combine for maximum net magnetization
   b. exhibit maximum saturation
   c. add vectorally to zero
   d. add vectorally to a maximum

☐ QUESTIONS TO PONDER

35. How many 3 mm slices can be obtained in 1inch when separated by a 0.5 mm interslice?

36. What are the two principle parameters governing spatial resolution?

37. What is the principal difference between 2D and 3D imaging?

38. How does image quality change with a change in the pixel/voxel size?

39. For what reason are magnetic field gradients interchanged?

Worksheet | 41

Pulse Sequence Diagrams

1. Of all the MRI pulse sequences, the simplest is probably:

    a. echo planar   c. inversion recovery
    b. fast spin echo   d. partial saturation

2. Which of the symbols in the figure below represents a 90^0 RF pulse?

    a. A   c. C
    b. B   d. D

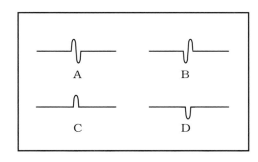

3. The number of multiple signals that are averaged is represented by:
    (1) SAR
    (2) Acq
    (3) FID
    (4) Nex

    a. 1, 2, and 3   c. 2 and 4
    b. 1 and 3   d. 4

4. An inversion recovery pulse sequence could not work with a single 180^0 RF pulse because:

    a. the resulting magnetization is overpowered by the B_0 field
    b. T2 relaxation would be too short
    c. T1 relaxation would be too short
    d. T2* relaxation would be too short

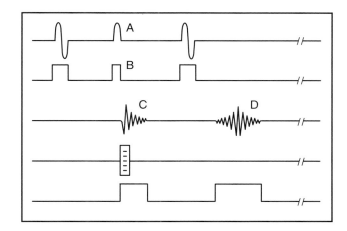

5. Which letter in the pulse sequence in the figure above represents a free induction decay?

    a. A   c. C
    b. B   d. D

6. Multiecho imaging in a conventional spin echo pulse sequence results in multiple sets of images having different:

    a. matrix size   c. contrast resolution
    b. field of view   d. spatial resolution

7. During a single TR of a partial saturation pulse sequence:

    a. an image can be constructed
    b. one line of the spatial frequency domain is measured
    c. one spin echo will be generated
    d. one gradient echo will be generated

8. What time is required to produce an image having a 256^2 matrix from two signal acquisitions with a repetition time of 2000 ms?

    a. 8.5 min   c. 25 min
    b. 17 min   d. 34 min

109

9. The principle advantage to multislice imaging is:

   a. multiple slices are imaged in the time necessary for one slice
   b. a different slice is imaged with each different phase-encoding gradient
   c. a different slice is imaged with each different frequency-encoding gradient
   d. several slices are imaged, each having a different image matrix

10. The purpose of the 90° RF pulse in an inversion recovery pulse sequence is to:

    a. lengthen T1 relaxation
    b. lengthen T2 relaxation
    c. lengthen T2* relaxation
    d. rotate the net magnetization onto the XY plane

11. Which letter in the following pulse sequence represents the frequency-encoding gradient?

    a. A   c. C
    b. B   d. D

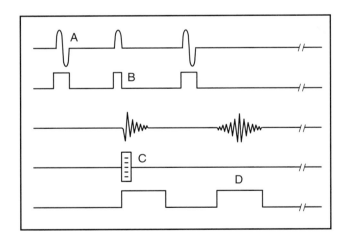

12. The time required for double echo imaging is _____ of that for single echo imaging.

    a. half   c. twice
    b. the same   d. four times

13. The MR signal observed in the partial saturation pulse sequence is:

    a. an FID
    b. a conventional spin echo
    c. a fast spin echo
    d. a gradient echo

14. What time is required to produce an image having a 128² matrix size from four signal acquisitions with a repetition time of 2200 ms?

    a. 4 min   c. 9.5 min
    b. 6 min   d. 19 min

15. Multislice imaging is possible because within one TR there occurs a different:
    (1) RF pulse
    (2) phase-encoding gradient
    (3) slice select gradient
    (4) frequency-encoding gradient

    a. 1, 2, and 3   c. 2 and 4
    b. 1 and 3   d. all are correct

16. The MR signal acquired during an inversion recovery pulse sequence is:

    a. an FID   c. a fast spin echo
    b. a spin echo   d. a gradient echo

17. Which letter in the following sequence represents a 90° RF pulse?

    a. A   c. C
    b. B   d. D

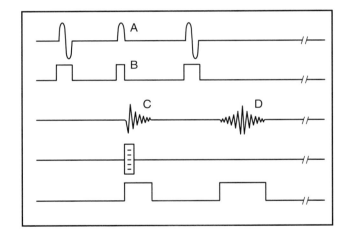

18. During the partial saturation pulse sequence the only change from one TR to the next is:

    a. the RF pulse
    b. the slice selection gradient
    c. the phase-encoding gradient
    d. the frequency-encoding gradient

19. MRI signals are averaged in order to:

    a. reduce imaging time
    b. improve contrast
    c. improve spatial resolution
    d. improve signal to noise ratio

110

20. The inversion recovery pulse sequence can be identified as:

    a. 90^0. . .90^0. . .90^0. . .90^0. . .
    b. 90^0. . .180^0. . .90^0. . .180^0. . .90^0. . .180^0. . .
    c. 180^0. . 180^0. . .180^0. . .180^0. . .
    d. 180^0. . .90^0. . .180^0. . .90^0. . .

21. Which letter in the pulse sequence in the following figure represents TE?

    a. A   c. C
    b. B   d. D

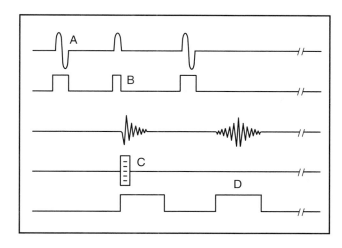

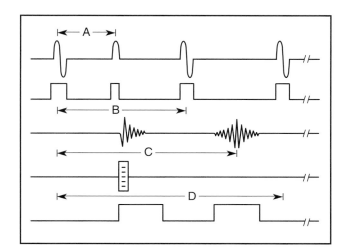

22. The conventional spin echo pulse sequence consists of

    a. 90^0. . .90^0. . .90^0. . .90^0. . .
    b. 90^0. . .180^0. . .90^0. . .180^0. . .90^0. . .180^0. . .
    c. 180^0. . 180^0. . .180^0. . .180^0. . .
    d. 180^0. . .90^0. . .180^0. . .90^0. . .

23. Which letter in the pulse sequence in the above figure represents a multiple pulsed phase–encoding gradient?

    a. A   c. C
    b. B   d. D

24. When MRI signals are averaged:

    a. imaging time is increased by the square root of the average
    b. imaging time is increased proportional with the number of averages
    c. noise is doubled
    d. noise is squared

25. The principle advantage of the inversion recovery pulse sequence is a:

    a. shorter imaging time
    b. larger field of view
    c. better contrast resolution
    d. better spatial resolution

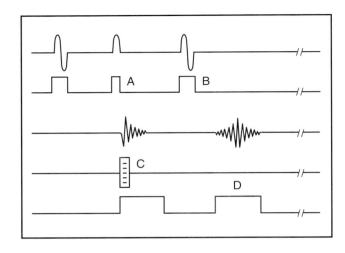

26. Which letter in the pulse sequence in the above figure represents the read gradient?

   a. A
   b. B
   c. C
   d. D

27. The time between the 90⁰ and 180⁰ RF pulse during spin echo imaging is:

   a. TR
   b. TR/2
   c. TE/2
   d. 2TE

28. If the number of signal acquisitions is doubled, the signal to noise ratio is:

   a. reduced to one half
   b. reduced to $1/\sqrt{2}$
   c. increased by $\sqrt{2}$
   d. doubled

29. The principle disadvantage of the inversion recovery pulse sequence is:

   a. longer imaging time
   b. smaller field of view
   c. worse contrast resolution
   d. worse spatial resolution

30. Which letter in the pulse sequence in the figure below represents inversion time?

   a. A
   b. B
   c. C
   d. D

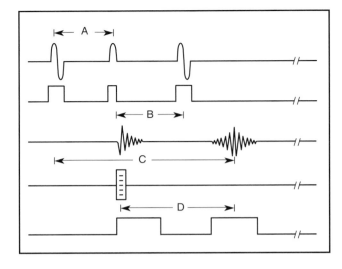

31. During a conventional spin echo pulse sequence, the free induction decay is:

   a. ignored
   b. doubled
   c. amplified
   d. inverted

32 A double echo, spin echo pulse sequence normally results in _____ images.

   a. T1- and T2-weighted
   b. T2- and spin density–weighted
   c. spin density– and T1-weighted
   d. T1-, T2-, and spin density–weighted

☐ **QUESTIONS TO PONDER**

33. What is the spin state and the signal amplitude at the mid-point of the spin echo?

34. Why is the frequency-encoding gradient referred to as the read gradient?

35. Why use a multiple spin echo technique?

36. Describe time of flight (TOF)?

37. What is phase contrast (PC)?

What is an Image?

1. An MR image would be identified as:

   a. abstract   c. visual
   b. imaginary   d. negative

2. Cones of the human retina:
   (1) are less sensitive to light than rods
   (2) are used primarily for photopic vision
   (3) can respond to intense light levels
   (4) are primarily used for daytime vision

   a. 1, 2, and 3   c. 2 and 4
   b. 1 and 3   d. all are correct

3. Match the following:
   1. intensity; 2. color; 3. day vision; 4. night vision

   a. brightness   _____
   b. scotopic vision   _____
   c. hue   _____
   d. photopic vision   _____

4. The character of a pixel is represented by its:
   (1) size
   (2) brightness
   (3) location
   (4) color

   a. 1, 2, and 3   c. 2 and 4
   b. 1 and 3   d. all are correct

5. Which of the following influence the character of
   an MRI pixel?
   (1) electron density
   (2) spin density
   (3) optical density
   (4) motion

   a. 1, 2, and 3   c. 2 and 4
   b. 1 and 3   d. all are correct

6. The visual receptors of the human eye include the:
   (1) cornea
   (2) rods
   (3) pupil
   (4) cones

   a. 1, 2, and 3   c. 2 and 4
   b. 1 and 3   d. all are correct

7. Rods of the human retina are:
   (1) more sensitive than cones
   (2) respond to intense light levels
   (3) used principally for scotopic vision
   (4) used primarily for daytime vision

   a. 1, 2, and 3   c. 2 and 4
   b. 1 and 3   d. 4 only is correct

8. Which letter in the above figure corresponds to
   a row of spins selected by the frequency-encoding
   gradient?

   a. A   c. C
   b. B   d. D

9. An MR image is sometimes called a _____ image.

    a. static
    b. dynamic
    c. representational
    d. characteristic

10. Human visual reception portrays light as:

    a. pixel location and character
    b. character and gray scale resolution
    c. gray scale resolution and intensity
    d. intensity and color

11. The ability to perceive fine detail is called:

    a. contrast perception
    b. visual acuity
    c. color perception
    d. conspiquity

12. The human eye can detect approximately _____ colors.

    a. two
    b. twenty
    c. two hundred
    d. two thousand

13. An MR image represents what tissue characteristic?

    a. optical density
    b. electron density
    c. gyromagnetic ratio
    d. hydrogen concentration

14. Match the following types of images with the appropriate image receptor:
    (1) scintillation detector; (2) film; (3) antenna; (4) piezoelectric crystal

    a. radiograph   _____
    b. ultrasonogram   _____
    c. radionuclide scan _____
    d. MR image   _____

15. Cones of the human retina are:

    a. concentrated at the center of the retina
    b. most numerous on the periphery of the retina
    c. all at the fovea centralis
    d. uniformly distributed on the retina

16. The ability to detect differences in brightness level is termed:

    a. contrast perception
    b. visual acuity
    c. color perception
    d. conspiquity

17. Pixels in an MR image have two characteristics:

    a. spatial resolution and contrast resolution
    b. contrast resolution and location
    c. location and character
    d. character and color

18. Match the following types of images with their representational media:
    (1) hydrogen concentration; (2) electron density; (3) reflectivity; (4) radioactive decay

    a. radiograph   _____
    b. ultrasonogram   _____
    c. radionuclide scan _____
    d. MR image   _____

19. Color is best visualized with:

    a. rods
    b. cones
    c. fovea centralis
    d. cornea

20. An MR image has two principle characteristics:

    a. spatial resolution and location
    b. location and character
    c. character and contrast resolution
    d. contrast resolution and spatial resolution

21. Which letter in the figure above represents a voxel?

    a. A
    b. B
    c. C
    d. D

22. The human eye can detect approximately _____ shades of gray.

    a. ten
    b. twenty
    c. forty
    d. eighty

☐ QUESTIONS TO PONDER

23. What are the three basic body planes?

24. How does bone marrow appear on an MR image?

25. How many shades of gray can we visualize?

26. How does magnification by reduced field of view (FOV) affect image quality?

Image Evaluation Criteria

1. When evaluating the gross anatomy visible in an MR image, the basic geometric factors are:
   (1) size
   (2) shape
   (3) position
   (4) character

   a. 1, 2, and 3   c. 2 and 4
   b. 1 and 3   d. all are correct

2. When evaluating the position of an anatomical structure in an MR image, the possibilities include:
   (1) normal
   (2) intrinsically malpositioned
   (3) extrinsically displaced
   (4) distorted

   a. 1, 2, and 3   c. 2 and 4
   b. 1 and 3   d. all are correct

3. Pixel location is determined by:

   a. intrinsic modification
   b. extrinsic pressure
   c. magnetic field gradients
   d. RF pulse sequence

4. The number of principle MR imaging parameters matches the number of primary colors. That number is:

   a. one   c. five
   b. three   d. seven

5. When evaluating the size of an anatomical part in an MR image, the specific descriptives are:
   (1) normal
   (2) intrinsically deformed
   (3) extrinsically compressed
   (4) distorted

   a. 1, 2, and 3   c. 2 and 4
   b. 1 and 3   d. all are correct

6. Abnormal tissue character is best exhibited by:

   a. intrinsic deformity
   b. extrinsic compression
   c. extrinsic displacement
   d. unexpected pixel brightness

7. When post-processing an MR image, ROI stands for:
   (1) region of interest
   (2) relaxation on inversion
   (3) a method of obtaining quantitative data
   (4) a method of observing qualitative change

   a. 1, 2, and 3   c. 2 and 4
   b. 1 and 3   d. 4

8. The principle parameters influencing the character is an MRI pixel are:
   (1) spin density
   (2) T1 relaxation
   (3) T2 relaxation
   (4) electromagnetic induction

   a. 1, 2, and 3   c. 2 and 4
   b. 1 and 3   d. all are correct

9. When evaluating the size of an anatomical structure in an MR image, the appropriate classifications are:
   (1) small
   (2) normal
   (3) large
   (4) distorted

   a. 1, 2, and 3   c. 2 and 4
   b. 1 and 3   d. all are correct

10. Which of the following seem to be easiest to detect on an MR image?

   a. diffuse abnormality
   b. diffuse pixel brightness
   c. focal lesion
   d. airway abnormality

11. Pixel character is determined by:

   a. intrinsic modification
   b. extrinsic pressure
   c. magnetic field gradients
   d. RF pulse sequence

12. Which of the diagrams in the figure below best represents T2 relaxation?

   a. A   c. C
   b. B   d. D

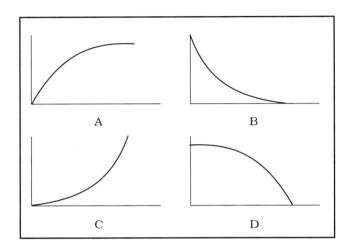

13. Why doesn't bone cause artifacts on MR images as it does on CT images?

14. How does cartilage appear on an MR image?

15. How many shades of gray would be on an ideal image?

16. Calculate the total scan time when the TR is 3000 ms, 2 NEX and 256 phase encoding steps are used.

17. What is the relationship of imaging time to T1 relaxation time?

Worksheet | **44**

MRI Character

1. The principle MRI parameters that affect pixel character are:
   (1) spin density
   (2) spin lattice relaxation time
   (3) spin spin relaxation time
   (4) electromagnetic induction

   a. 1, 2, and 3   c. 2 and 4
   b. 1 and 3   d. all are correct

2. One reason that pure spin density images, T1 images, or T2 images are not obtained is:

   a. it requires imager modifications
   b. it takes too long
   c. it costs too much
   d. it cannot be done

Questions 3 through 10 refer to the following figure.

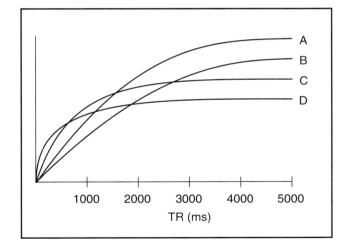

3. Which tissue has highest equilibrium magnetization?

   a. A   c. C
   b. B   d. D

4. Which tissue has the shortest relaxation time?

   a. A   c. C
   b. B   d. D

5. At what approximate TR is the longitudinal magnetization for tissues B and C equal?

   a. 500 ms   c. 2500
   b. 1500 ms   d. 3500

6. At a TR of 500 ms which tissue should appear brightest?

   a. A   c. C
   b. B   d. D

7. At a TR of 2000 ms which tissue should appear darkest?

   a. A   c. C
   b. B   d. D

8. At a TR of 2000 ms which of the following tissues has reached equilibrium?
   (1) A
   (2) B
   (3) C
   (4) D

   a. 1, 2, and 3   c. 2 and 4
   b. 1 and 3   d. 4

9. At a TR of 1000 ms which of the tissues is most saturated?
   (1) A
   (2) B
   (3) C
   (4) D

   a. 1, 2, and 3   c. 2 and 4
   b. 1 and 3   d. all are correct

10. If a TR of approximately 1200 ms is chosen, which tissues will exhibit the lowest contrast?

    a. A/B   c. C/D
    b. B/C   d. D/A

11. When considering brain tissue, rank gray matter (GM), white matter (WM) and cerebral spinal fluid (CSF) in increasing order of net magnetization at equilibrium.

    a. GM, WM, CSF   c. WM, GM, CSF
    b. GM, CSF, WM   d. WM, CSF, GM

12. When considering brain tissue, rank GM, WM and CSF in increasing order of spin lattice relaxation time.

    a. GM, WM, CSF   c. WM, GM, CSF
    b. GM, CSF, WM   d. WM, CSF, GM

13. A partial saturation image made with a short repetition time is most likely a (an):

    a. spin density–weighted image
    b. T1-weighted image
    c. T2-weighted image
    d. a pure image

14. In a conventional spin echo pulse sequence, following the 90° RF pulse:
    (1) $M_{xy} = 0$
    (2) $M_{xy} = M_0$
    (3) $M_z = M_0$
    (4) $M_z = 0$

    a. 1, 2, and 3   c. 2 and 4
    b. 1 and 3   d. 4

Questions 15 through 18 refer to the following figure.

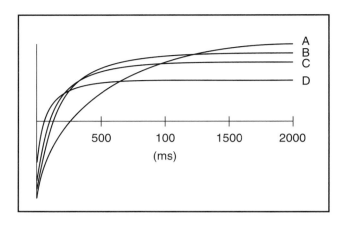

15. The relaxation shown is:

    a. spin density relaxation
    b. spin lattice relaxation
    c. spin spin relaxation
    d. pure image relaxation

16. Which of the four tissues has the lowest magnetization at equilibrium?

    a. A   c. C
    b. B   d. D

17. Which of the four tissues has the longest relaxation time?

    a. A   c. C
    b. B   d. D

18. At approximately 1000 ms which tissue should appear brightest?

    a. A   c. C
    b. B   d. D

19. In a partial saturation pulse sequence:

    a. all FIDs are of equal amplitude
    b. all spin echoes are of equal amplitude
    c. early FIDs have a higher amplitude
    d. early spin echoes have higher amplitude

20. The principle secondary MRI parameters that affect pixel character are:
    (1) chemical shift
    (2) paramagnetic materials
    (3) magnetic susceptibility
    (4) motion

    a. 1, 2, and 3   c. 2 and 4
    b. 1 and 3   d. all are correct

21. Rank the intrinsic contrast of the MRI parameters for soft tissues (lowest to highest contrast):

    a. spin density, spin lattice relaxation time, spin spin relaxation time
    b. spin lattice relaxation time, spin spin relaxation time, spin density
    c. spin spin relaxation time, spin density, spin lattice relaxation time
    d. spin lattice relaxation time, spin density, spin spin relaxation time

22. In a partial saturation pulse sequence, after a 90^0 RF pulse:
    (1) $M_{xy} = 0$
    (2) $M_{xy} = M_0$
    (3) $M_z = M_0$
    (4) $M_z = 0$

    a. 1, 2, and 3   c. 2 and 4
    b. 1 and 3   d. 4

23. Inversion recovery pulse sequences are employed principally to obtain

    a. spin density-weighted images
    b. T1-weighted images
    c. T2-weighted images
    d. a pure image

Questions 24 through 28 refer to the pulse sequence shown in the following figure.

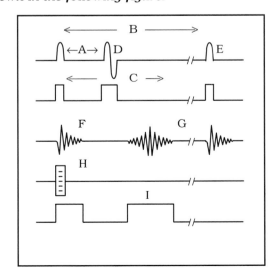

24. The echo time is:

    a. A   c. C
    b. B   d. D

25. The repetition time is:

    a. A   c. C
    b. B   d. D

26. The RF refocussing pulse is:

    a. A   c. C
    b. B   d. D

27. The FID is:

    a. D   c. F
    b. E   d. G

28. The spin echo is:

    a. F   c. H
    b. G   D. I

29. In a conventional spin echo pulse sequence, following the 180^0 RF pulse:

    a. $M_{xy} = 0$ c. $M_z = 0$
    b. $M_{xy} = M_0$ d. $M_z = M_0$

30. Match the approximate percent contrast difference of soft tissues with the appropriate imaging parameter.
    (1) 5%; (2) 15%; (3) 25%; (4) 35%

    a. spin spin relaxation time   ____
    b. spin lattice relaxation time ____
    c. spin density   ____
    d. attenuation coefficient   ____

31. The spin spin relaxation time is measured:

    a. by a 0 to 100 relative scale
    b. with hydrogen units (HU) from -1000 to +1000
    c. in 10's of milliseconds
    d. in 100's of milliseconds

32. Which of the following pulse sequences results in a weighted MR image?
    (1) partial saturation
    (2) inversion recovery
    (3) spin echo
    (4) gradient echo

    a. 1, 2, and 3   c. 2 and 4
    b. 1 and 3   d. all are correct

Questions 33 through 37 refer to the following figure.

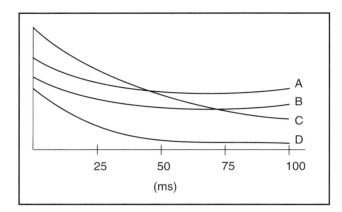

33. Which of the four tissues has the shortest relaxation time?

    a. A   c. C
    b. B   d. D

34. Which of the four tissues has the highest net magnetization at equilibrium?

    a. A   c. C
    b. B   d. D

35. This is a graph of:

    a. spin density vs relaxation time
    b. spin density vs time
    c. M_z vs time
    d. M_{xy} vs time

36. At a TE of 100 ms which tissue should appear brightest?

    a. A   c. C
    b. B   d. D

37. At a TE of 25 ms which tissue should appear brightest?

    a. A   c. C
    b. B   d. D

38. Following the first 180° RF pulse in an inversion recovery pulse sequence:
    (1) $M_z = 0$ (2) $M_{xy} = 0$ (3) $M_z = M_0$ (4) $M_z = -M_0$

    a. 1, 2, and 3   c. 2 and 4
    b. 1 and 3   d. 4

39. Following the 90° RF pulse in an inversion recovery pulse sequence:

    a. $M_z = 0$ c. $M_z = -M_0$
    b. $M_z = M_0$ d. $M_{xy} = 0$

Questions 40 through 43 refer to the following figure.

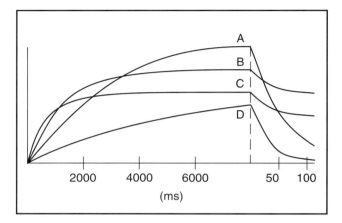

40. At a TR of 10,000 ms and a TE of 100 ms, which tissue should appear brightest?

    a. A   c. C
    b. B   d. D

41. Which tissue has the shortest T1 relaxation time?

    a. A   c. C
    b. B   d. D

42. Which tissue has the shortest T2 relaxation time?

    a. A   c. C
    b. B   d. D

43. Which tissue has the highest net magnetization at equilibrium?

    a. A   c. C
    b. B   d. D

44. The Houndsfield scale as used in CT has a range of

    a. 0 to 100%   c. -500 to +500
    b. 0 to 1000%   d. -1000 to +1000

45. One relationship between spin spin relaxation time (T2) and spin lattice relaxation time (T1) is:

   a. T2 ≤ T1   c. T2 > T1
   b. T2 < T1   d. T2 ≥ T1

46. The term saturation in partial saturation pulse sequence means:
   (1) $M_{xy} = 0$
   (2) $M_{xy} = M_0$
   (3) $M_z = M_0$
   (4) $M_z = 0$

   a. 1, 2, and 3   c. 2 and 4
   b. 1 and 3   d. 4

47. The image resulting from a partial saturation pulse sequence is:

   a. a pure image
   b. a spin density–weighted image
   c. a T1-weighted image
   d. a T2-weighted image

Questions 48 through 51 refer to the following figure.

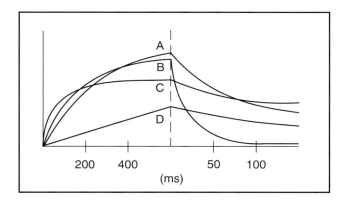

48. At a TR of 10,000 ms and a TE of 100 ms, which tissue should appear brightest?

   a. A   c. C
   b. B   d. D

49. Which tissue has the shortest T1 relaxation time?

   a. A   c. C
   b. B   d. D

50. Which tissue has the shortest T2 relaxation time?

   a. A   c. C
   b. B   d. D

51. Which tissue has the highest net magnetization at equilibrium?

   a. A   c. C
   b. B   d. D

52. The spin density of various tissues is measured:

   a. by a 0 to 100 relative scale
   b. with hydrogen units (HU) from -1000 to +1000
   c. in 10's of milliseconds
   d. in 100's of milliseconds

53. When MR images are rendered in color the primary colors employed are:

   a. blue, green, and yellow
   b. green, yellow, and red
   c. red, blue, and yellow
   d. blue, green, and red

54. For saturated spins to fully relax to equilibrium:

   a. the TE must equal the TR
   b. the TE must exceed the TR
   c. the TE must equal five T1
   d. the TR must equal five T1

55. The spin lattice relaxation time is measured:

   a. by a 0 to 100 relative scale
   b. with hydrogen units (HU) from -1000 to +1000
   c. in 10's of milliseconds
   d. in 100's of milliseconds

Questions 56 through 59 refer to the following figure.

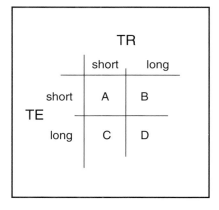

56. Which letter represents the spin echo pulse sequence combination of TR and TE that will result in a spin density–weighted image?

   a. A   c. C
   b. B   d. D

57. Which letter represents the spin echo pulse sequence combination of TR and TE that will result in a T1-weighted image?

   a. A
   b. B

   c. C
   d. D

58. Which letter represents the spin echo pulse sequence combination of TR and TE that will result in a T2-weighted image?

   a. A
   b. B

   c. C
   d. D

☐ QUESTIONS TO PONDER

59. What does hypointense mean?

60. What type of image is considered more anatomical than pathological?

61. What is the relationship between signal intensity and image contrast?

62. How does a low signal-to-noise ratio (S/N) image appear?

SECTION III

Imaging Procedures

Worksheet | 45

Head—Sagittal Plane

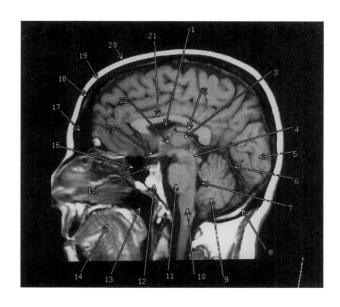

Questions 1 to 24 refer to the figure above.

1. What type of contrast is dominant in this sagittal image?

   a. spin density   c. T2
   b. T1   d. T2*

2. Which arrow points to the cerebellum? _____

3. Which arrow points to the cerebral Aqueduct of Sylvius? _____

4. Which arrow points to the clivus? _____

5. Which arrow points to the corpus callosum? _____

6. Which arrow points to the diploic space of frontal bone? _____

7. Which arrow points to the fornix? _____

8. Which arrow points to the fourth ventricle? _____

9. Which arrow points to the frontal sinus? _____

10. Which arrow points to the lateral ventricle? _____

11. Which arrow points to the medulla oblongata? _____

12. Which arrow points to the nasopharynx? _____

13. Which arrow points to the occipital bone? _____

14. Which arrow points to the occipital lobe? _____

15. Which arrow points to the optic chiasm? _____

16. Which arrow points to the outer table of frontal bone? _____

17. Which arrow points to the pituitary gland? _____

18. Which arrow points to the pons? _____

19. Which arrow points to the scalp? _____

20. Which arrow points to the sphenoid sinus? _____

21. Which arrow points to the tentorium? _____

22. Which arrow points to the thalamus? _____

23. Which arrow points to the third ventricle? _____

24. Which arrow points to the tongue? _____

Questions 25 to 33 refer to the figure below.

25. Which type of contrast is dominant in this sagittal image?

    a. spin density   c. T2
    b. T1   d. T2*

26. Which arrow points to the cerebellum? _____

27. Which arrow points to the lateral rectus muscle? _____

28. Which arrow points to the lateral ventricle? _____

29. Which arrow points to the maxillary sinus? _____

30. Which arrow points to the optic nerve? _____

31. Which arrow points to the orbital fat? _____

32. Which arrow points to the superior rectus muscle? _____

33. Which arrow points to the temporal lobe? _____

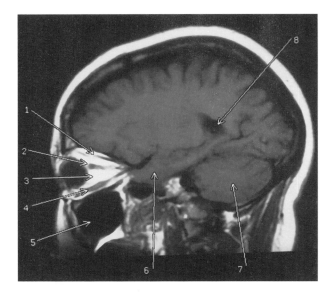

Worksheet 46

Head—Transverse Plane

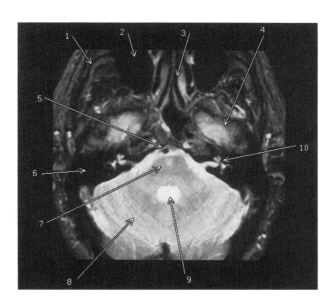

Questions 1 to 12 refer to the figure above.

1. What type of contrast is dominant in this image?

   a. spin density   c. T2
   b. T1   d. T2*

2. Which arrow points to the basilar artery? _____

3. Which arrow points to the cerebellum? _____

4. Which arrow points to the fourth ventricle? _____

5. Which arrow points to the internal auditory canal? _____

6. Which arrow points to the maxillary sinus? _____

7. Which arrow points to the nasal turbinate? _____

8. Which arrow points to the pons? _____

9. Which arrow points to the temporal bone? _____

10. Which arrow points to the temporal lobe? _____

11. Which arrow points to the zygomatic arch? _____

12. What four separate nerves enter the internal auditory canal?

Questions 13 to 26 refer to the following figure.

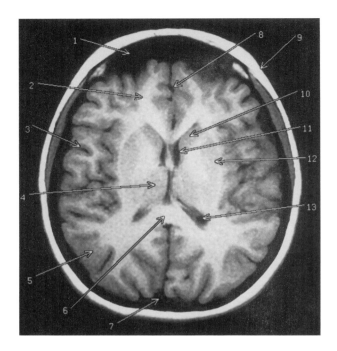

13. What type of contrast is dominant in this image?

    a. spin density   c. T2
    b. T1   d. T2*

14. Which arrow points to the basal ganglia? _____

15. Which arrow points to the caudate nucleus? _____

16. Which arrow points to the frontal horn of lateral ventricle? _____

17. Which arrow points to the frontal sinus? _____

18. Which arrow points to the gray matter? _____

19. Which arrow points to the interhemispheric fissure? _____

20. Which arrow points to the scalp? _____

21. Which arrow points to the splenium of the corpus callosum? _____

22. Which arrow points to the sulcus? _____

23. Which arrow points to the superior sagittal sinus? _____

24. Which arrow points to the thalamus? _____

25. Which arrow points to the trigone of lateral ventricle? _____

26. Which arrow points to the white matter? _____

Questions 27 to 34 refer to the figure below.

27. What type of contrast is dominant in this image?

    a. spin density   c. T2
    b. T1   d. T2*

28. Which arrow points to the caudate nucleus? _____

29. Which arrow points to the corpus callosum? _____

30. Which arrow points to the CSF in sulci? _____

31. Which arrow points to the gray matter? _____

32. Which arrow points to the lateral ventricle? _____

33. Which arrow points to the scalp? _____

34. Which arrow points to the white matter? _____

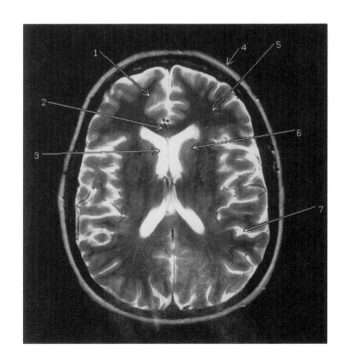

Worksheet 47

Head—Coronal Plane

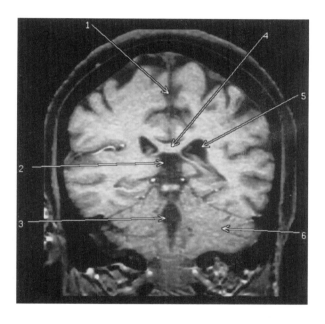

Questions 1 to 6 refer to the figure above.

1. Which arrow points to the cerebellum? _____

2. Which arrow points to the corpus callosum? _____

3. Which arrow points to the falx cerebri? _____

4. Which arrow points to the fourth ventricle? _____

5. Which arrow points to the lateral ventricle? _____

6. Which arrow points to the third ventricle? _____

Questions 7 to 19 refer to the figure to the right .

7. What type of pulse sequence was most likely used to create this coronal image?

    a. fast spin echo   c. inversion recovery
    b. gradient echo   d. spin echo

8. Which arrow points to the corpus callosum? _____

9. Which arrow points to the internal carotid artery? _____

10. Which arrow points to the lateral ventricle? _____

11. Which arrow points to the mandibular condyle? _____

12. Which arrow points to the optic chiasm? _____

13. Which arrow points to the pituitary gland? _____

14. Which arrow points to the pituitary infundibulum? _____

15. Which arrow points to the sphenoid sinus? _____

16. Which arrow points to the Sylvian fissure? _____

17. Which arrow points to the temporal lobe? _____

18. Which arrow points to the white matter? _____

19. What cavity is located immediately superior to the optic chiasm?

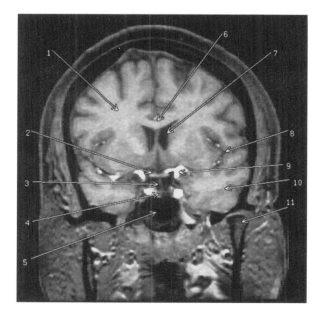

20. What type of contrast is dominant in the two preceding figures?

    a. spin density   c. T2
    b. T1   d. T2*

21. What type of pulse sequence was most likely used to create these coronal images?

    a. fast spin echo   c. inversion recovery
    b. gradient echo   d. spin echo

Worksheet 48

Vascular Neck

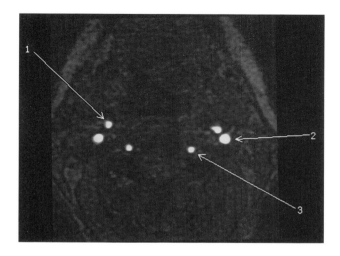

Questions 1 to 5 refer to the figure above.

1. In order to show only the arterial flow in this image, how are saturation bands placed in relation to the area of interest?

   a. anterior   c. posterior
   b. inferior   d. superior

2. Which arrow points to the external carotid artery?
   _____

3. Which arrow points to the internal carotid artery?
   _____

4. Which arrow points to the vertebral artery? _____

5. For MR angiography, what pulse sequence technique is based on the entry slice phenomenon?

Questions 6 to 10 refer to the figure below.

6. Which arrow points to the internal carotid artery?
   _____

7. Which arrow points to the external carotid artery?
   _____

8. Which arrow points to the common carotid artery?
   _____

9. Which arrow points to the vertebral artery? _____

10. The left vertebral artery branches off which great vessel?

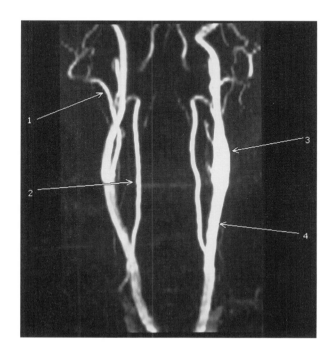

131

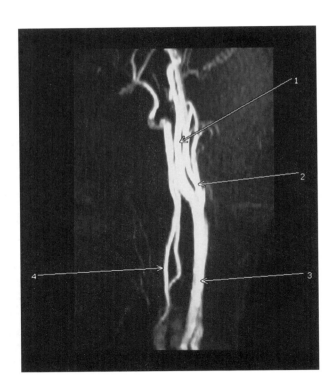

Questions 11 to 15 refer to the figure above.

11. Which arrow points to the external carotid artery? _____

12. Which arrow points to the vertebral artery? _____

13. Which arrow points to the internal carotid artery? _____

14. Which arrow points to the common carotid artery? _____

15. The right common carotid artery branches off which great vessel?

Worksheet | 49

Vascular Head

Questions 1 to 6 refer to the figure below.

1. The vasculature in this image is projected into which plane?

   a. transverse   c. sagittal
   b. coronal   d. oblique

2. Which arrow points to the anterior cerebral artery? _____

3. Which arrow points to the anterior communicating artery? _____

4. Which arrow points to the basilar artery? _____

5. Which arrow points to the internal carotid artery? _____

6. Which arrow points to the middle cerebral artery? _____

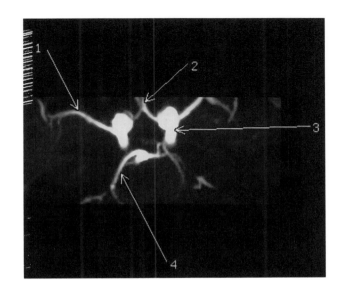

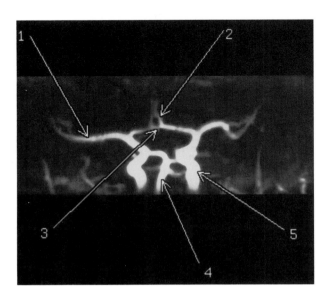

Questions 7 to 11 refer to the figure above.

7. The vasculature in this image is projected into which plane?

   a. transverse   c. sagittal
   b. coronal   d. oblique

8. Which arrow points to the anterior cerebral artery? _____

9. Which arrow points to the internal carotid artery? _____

10. Which arrow points to the middle cerebral artery? _____

11. Which arrow points to the posterior cerebral artery? _____

Questions 12 to 15 refer to the following figure.

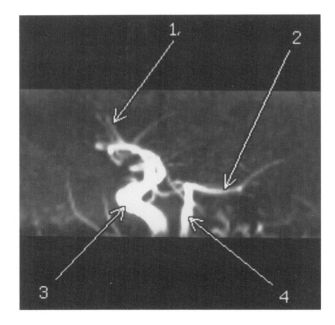

12. Which arrow points to the anterior cerebral artery? _____

13. Which arrow points to the basilar artery? _____

14. Which arrow points to the internal carotid artery? _____

15. Which arrow points to the posterior cerebral artery? _____

C-Spine—Sagittal Plane

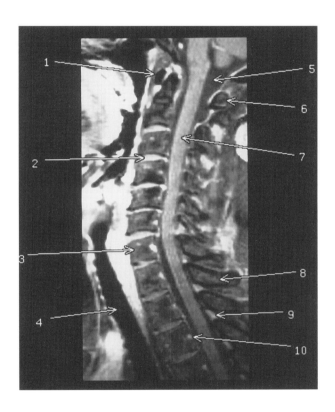

Questions 1 to 9 refer to the figure above.

1. Which arrow points to the anterior arch of C1? ____

2. Which arrow points to the epidural fat? ____

3. Which arrow points to the posterior arch of C1? ____

4. Which arrow points to the spinal cord? ____

5. Which arrow points to the spinous process? ____

6. Which arrow points to the subarachnoid space? ____

7. Which arrow points to the trachea? ____

8. Arrow #2 indicates which intervertebral space? ____

9. Arrow #3 indicates which vertebral body? ____

Questions 10 to 16 refer to the figure below.

10. What type of contrast is dominant in this image?

    a. spin density   c. T2
    b. T1   d. T2*

11. Arrow #1 indicates which cervical vertebra? _____

12. Arrow #2 indicates which intervertebral disc space? _____

13. Arrow #3 indicates which vertebral body? _____

14. Arrow #4 indicates the _____.

15. Arrow #5 indicates the _____.

16. Arrow #6 indicates the _____.

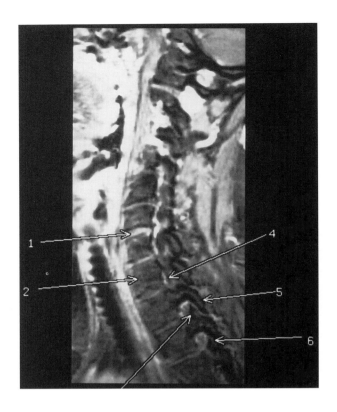

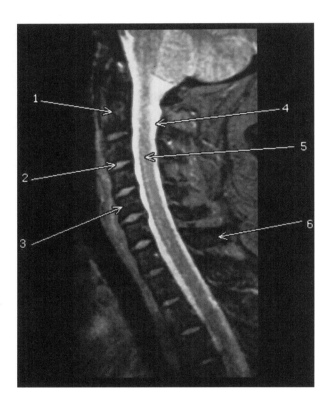

Questions 17 to 23 refer to the above figure.

17. Which arrow points to the facet joint? _____

18. Which arrow points to the inferior facet? _____

19. Which arrow points to the intervertebral disc? _____

20. Which arrow points to the neural foramen? _____

21. Which arrow points to the superior facet? _____

22. Which arrow points to the vertebral body? _____

23. Through what bony structure do the nerve roots exit? _____.

C-Spine—Transverse and Coronal Planes

Questions 1 to 6 refer to the figure below.

1. What type of contrast is dominant in this image?

   a. spin density   c. T2
   b. T1   d. T2*

2. Which arrow points to the epidural fat? _____

3. Which arrow points to the lamina? _____

4. Which arrow points to the nerve root? _____

5. Which arrow points to the spinal cord? _____

6. Which arrow points to the subarachnoid space?

   _____

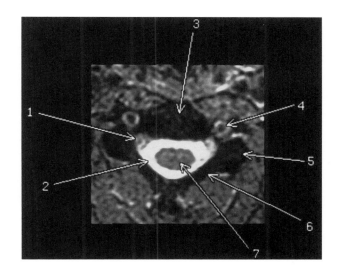

Questions 7 to 15 refer to the above figure.

7. What type of contrast is dominant in this image?

   a. spin density   c. T2
   b. T1   d. T2*

8. Which arrow points to the cerebrospinal fluid?
   _____

9. Which arrow points to the facet? _____

10. Which arrow points to the lamina? _____

11. Which arrow points to the neural foramen? _____

12. Which arrow points to the spinal cord? _____

13. Which arrow points to the vertebral artery? _____

14. Which arrow points to the vertebral body? _____

15. Through what structure does the vertebral artery
    pass? _____.

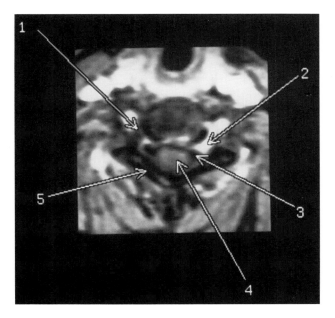

Questions 16 to 23 refer to the following figure.

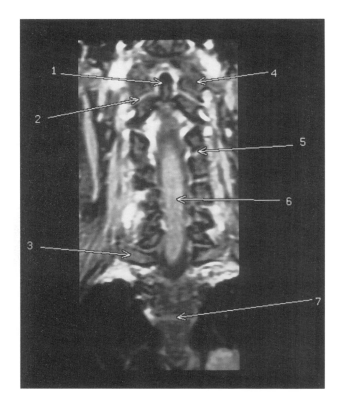

16. What is the name of the joint space indicated by arrow #2? _____.

17. Which arrow points to the facet joint? _____

18. Which arrow points to the intervertebral disc? _____

19. Which arrow points to the lateral mass of C1? _____

20. Which arrow points to the odontoid process? _____

21. Which arrow points to the rib? _____

22. Which arrow points to the spinal cord? _____

23. The neural foramen is formed by what bony segments? _____

Worksheet | 52

T-Spine

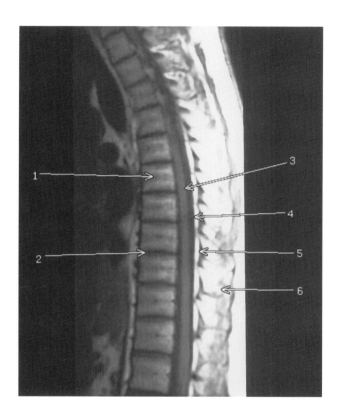

Questions 1 to 7 refer to the figure above.

1. What type of contrast is dominant in this image?

   a. spin density   c. T2
   b. T1   d. T2*

2. Which arrow points to the epidural fat? _____

3. Which arrow points to the intervertebral disc?

   _____

4. Which arrow points to the spinal cord? _____

5. Which arrow points to the spinous process? _____

6. Which arrow points to the subarachnoid space?

   _____

7. Which arrow points to the vertebral body? _____

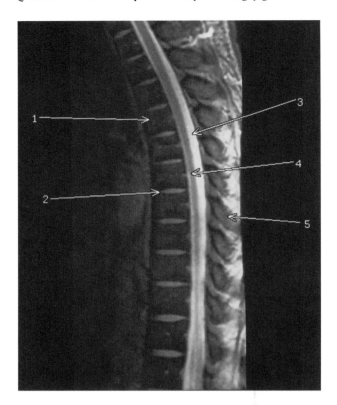

8. What type of contrast is dominant in this image?

    a. spin density   c. T2
    b. T1   d. T2*

9. With this image contrast, the discs normally have a relatively strong signal due to what factor?

10. Which arrow points to the intervertebral disc? _____

11. Which arrow points to the spinal cord? _____

12. Which arrow points to the spinous process? _____

13. Which arrow points to the subarachnoid space? _____

14. Which arrow points to the vertebral body? _____

15. Which arrow points to the facet joint? _____

16. Which arrow points to the inferior facet? _____

17. Which arrow points to the intervertebral disc? _____

18. Which arrow points to the nerve root? _____

19. Which arrow points to the pedicle? _____

20. Which arrow points to the superior facet? _____

21. Which arrow points to the vertebral body? _____

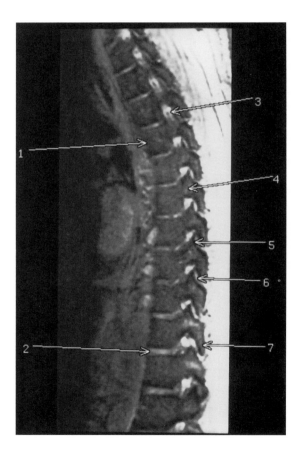

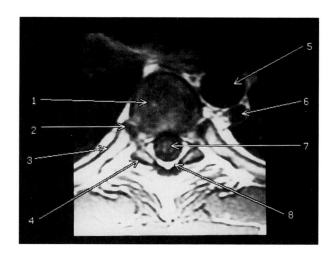

Questions 22 to 30 refer to the above figure.

22. What type of contrast is dominant in this image?

    a. spin density   c. T2
    b. T1   d. T2*

23. Which arrow points to the aorta? _____

24. Which arrow points to the azygos? _____

25. Which arrow points to the costovertebral joint space? _____

26. Which arrow points to the epidural fat? _____

27. Which arrow points to the intervertebral disc? _____

28. Which arrow points to the lamina? _____

29. Which arrow points to the rib? _____

30. Which arrow points to the spinal cord? _____

Worksheet   53

L-Spine—Sagittal Plane

Questions 1 to 8 refer to the following figure .

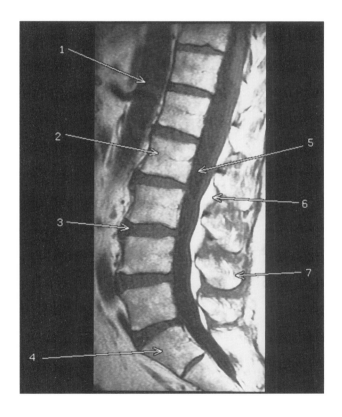

1. What type of contrast is dominant in this image?

   a. spin density   c. T2
   b. T1   d. T2*

2. Which arrow points to the aorta? _____

3. Which arrow points to the epidural fat? _____

4. Which arrow points to the spinous process? _____

5. Which arrow points to the subarachnoid space? _____

6. Which intervertebral disc space is indicated by arrow #3? _____

7. Which vertebral body is indicated by arrow #2? _____

8. Which vertebral body is indicated by arrow #4? _____

Questions 9 to 16 refer to the figure below.

9. What type of contrast is dominant in this image?

    a. spin density   c. T2
    b. T1   d. T2*

10. Which vertebral body is indicated by arrow #1?

    _____

11. Which intervertebral disc is indicated by arrow #2?

    _____

12. Which vertebral body is indicated by arrow #3?

    _____

13. Which arrow points to the cauda equina? _____

14. Which arrow points to the cerebrospinal fluid?

    _____

15. Which arrow points to the conus medullaris? _____

16. Which arrow points to the spinous process? _____

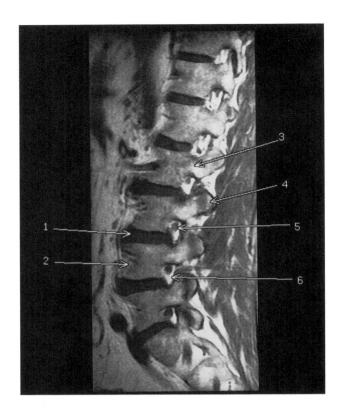

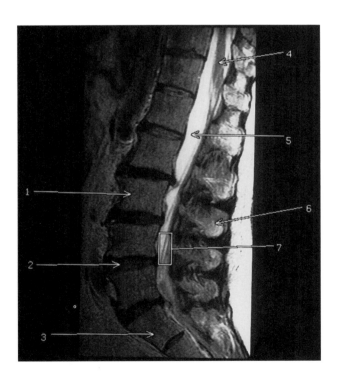

Questions 17 to 22 refer to the above figure.

17. Which arrow points to the articulating process?

    _____

18. Which arrow points to the epidural fat? _____

19. Which arrow points to the intervertebral disc?

    _____

20. Which arrow points to the nerve root? _____

21. Which arrow points to the pedicle? _____

22. Which arrow points to the vertebral body? _____

L-Spine—Transverse Plane

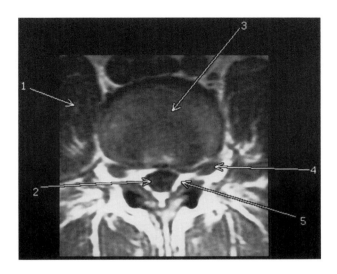

Questions 7 to 14 refer to the figure below.

7. Which arrow points to the epidural fat? _____

8. Which arrow points to the inferior facet? _____

9. Which arrow points to the intervertebral disc? _____

10. Which arrow points to the nerve root? _____

11. Which arrow points to the psoas muscle? _____

12. Which arrow points to the spinal canal? _____

13. Which arrow points to the spinous process? _____

14. Which arrow points to the superior facet? _____

Questions 1 to 6 refer to the above figure.

1. What type of contrast is dominant in this image?

    a. spin density   c. T2
    b. T1   d. T2*

2. Which arrow points to the epidural fat? _____

3. Which arrow points to the nerve root? _____

4. Which arrow points to the psoas muscle? _____

5. Which arrow points to the spinal canal? _____

6. Which arrow points to the vertebral body? _____

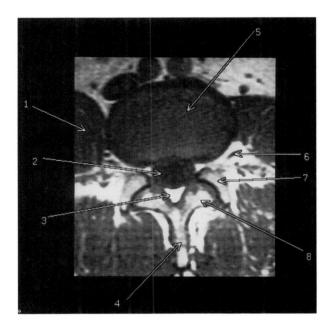

Questions 15 to 22 refer to the following figure.

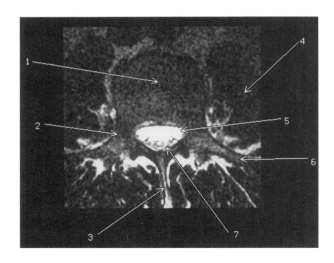

15. What type of contrast is dominant in this image?

    a. spin density   c. T2
    b. T1   d. T2*

16. Which arrow points to the cerebrospinal fluid? _____

17. Which arrow points to the nerve root? _____

18. Which arrow points to the pedicle? _____

19. Which arrow points to the psoas muscle? _____

20. Which arrow points to the spinous process? _____

21. Which arrow points to the transverse process? _____

22. Which arrow points to the vertebral body? _____

Questions 23 to 30 refer to the figure below.

23. What type of contrast is dominant in this image?

    a. spin density   c. T2
    b. T1   d. T2*

24. Which arrow points to the cauda equina? _____

25. Which arrow points to the cerebrospinal fluid? _____

26. Which arrow points to the epidural fat? _____

27. Which arrow points to the inferior facet? _____

28. Which arrow points to the intervertebral disc? _____

29. Which arrow points to the nerve root? _____

30. Which arrow points to the spinous process? _____

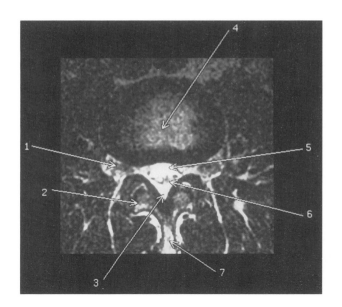

Worksheet 55

Chest—Transverse Plane

Questions 1 to 7 refer to the following figure.

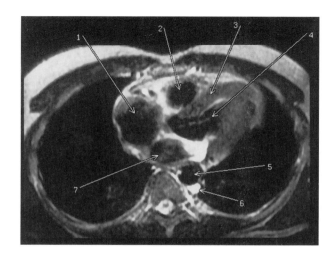

Questions 8 to 15 refer to the figure below.

8. Which arrow points to the descending aorta? _____

9. Which arrow points to the hemiazygos vein? _____

10. Which arrow points to the left atrium? _____

11. Which arrow points to the left ventricle? _____

12. Which arrow points to the right ventricle? _____

13. Which arrow points to the root of aorta? _____

14. Which arrow points to the sternum? _____

15. Which arrow points to the superior vena cava?

_____

1. Which arrow points to the aorta? _____

2. Which arrow points to the hemiazygos vein? _____

3. Which arrow points to the interventricular septum? _____

4. Which arrow points to the left atrium? _____

5. Which arrow points to the left ventricle? _____

6. Which arrow points to the right atrium? _____

7. Which arrow points to the right ventricle? _____

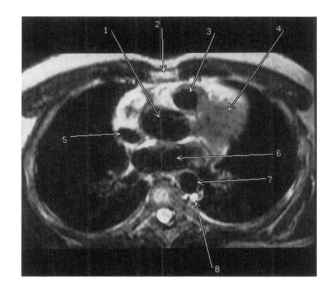

Questions 16 to 18 refer to the two preceding figures.

16. Which of the preceding two images through the heart is the most inferior slice?

17. Which of the four heart chambers is located most anteriorly?

    a. left ventricle
    b. right ventricle
    c. left atrium
    d. right atrium

18. Which of the four heart chambers is located most posteriorly?

    a. left ventricle
    b. right ventricle
    c. left atrium
    d. right atrium

Worksheet | 56

Chest—Coronal Plane

Questions 1 to 8 refer to the figure below.

1. Which arrow points to the aortic arch? _____

2. Which arrow points to the inferior vena cava? _____

3. Which arrow points to the left atrium? _____

4. Which arrow points to the left main bronchus? _____

5. Which arrow points to the liver? _____

6. Which arrow points to the rib? _____

7. Which arrow points to the right main bronchus? _____

8. Which arrow points to the upper lobe? _____

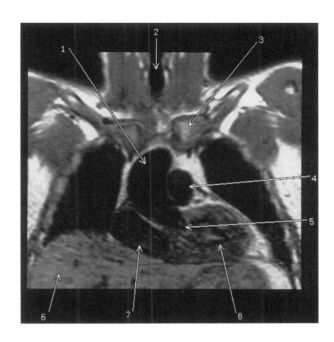

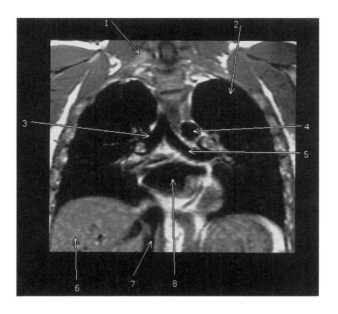

Questions 9 to 17 refer to the above figure.

9. Which arrow points to the aorta? _____

10. Which arrow points to the aortic valve? _____

11. Which arrow points to the clavicle? _____

12. Which arrow points to the left ventricle? _____

13. Which arrow points to the liver? _____

14. Which arrow points to the pulmonary artery? _____

15. Which arrow points to the right atrium? _____

16. Which arrow points to the trachea? _____

17. During which phase of the cardiac cycle would the luminal capacity of the left ventricle be at its greatest?

18. Which of the preceding two coronal images through the heart is the most anterior slice?

Worksheet 57

Chest-Sagittal Plane

Questions 1 to 9 refer to the figure below.

1. Which arrow points to the ascending aorta? _____

2. Which arrow points to the esophagus? _____

3. Which arrow points to the left atrium? _____

4. Which arrow points to the liver? _____

5. Which arrow points to the manubrium? _____

6. Which arrow points to the right pulmonary artery? _____

7. Which arrow points to the right ventricle? _____

8. Which arrow points to the sternum? _____

9. Which arrow points to the trachea? _____

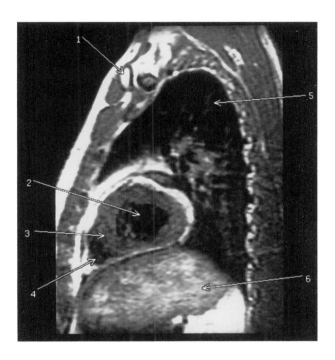

Questions 10 to 15 refer to the figure above.

10. Which arrow points to the clavicle? _____

11. Which arrow points to the interventricular septum? _____

12. Which arrow points to the left ventricle? _____

13. Which arrow points to the liver? _____

14. Which arrow points to the lung? _____

15. Which arrow points to the right ventricle? _____

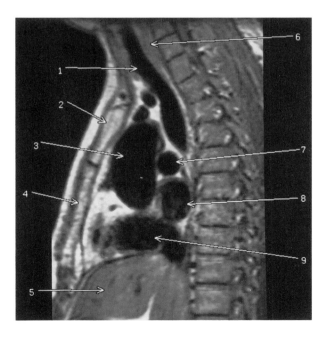

Worksheet 58

Breast

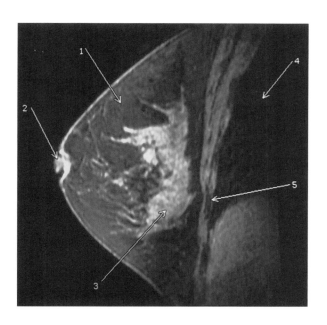 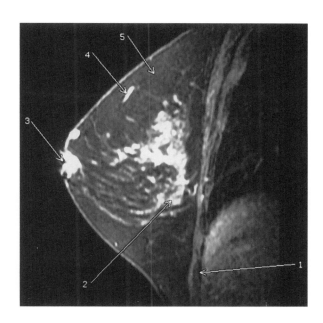

Questions 1 to 5 refer to the first figure above.

1. Which arrow points to the breast parenchyma? _____

2. Which arrow points to the fatty tissue? _____

3. Which arrow points to the lung field? _____

4. Which arrow points to the nipple? _____

5. Which arrow points to the rib? _____

Questions 6 to 10 refer to the second figure above.

6. Which arrow points to the blood vessel? _____

7. Which arrow points to the breast parenchyma? _____

8. Which arrow points to the fatty tissue? _____

9. Which arrow points to the nipple? _____

10. Which arrow points to the rib? _____

Questions 11 and 12 refer to both of the above figures.

11. Which of the two images demonstrates contrast enhancement?

    a. the first figure   b. the second figure

12. On the post-contrast image, why would RF spoiling be utilized?

Questions 13 to 18 refer to the first figure below.

13. Which arrow points to the breast parenchyma? _____

14. Which arrow points to the chest wall? _____

15. Which arrow points to the fatty tissue? _____

16. Which arrow points to the lung field? _____

17. Which arrow points to the nipple? _____

18. Which arrow points to the silicone implant? _____

Questions 19 to 22 refer to the second figure below.

19. Which arrow points to the breast parenchyma? _____

20. Which arrow points to the fatty tissue? _____

21. Which arrow points to the nipple? _____

22. Which arrow points to the silicone implant? _____

23. Which image demonstrates fat suppression?

    a. the first figure   b. the second figure

24. In what imaging plane is the breast anatomy demonstrated in the figures on this and the preceding page?

    a. transverse   c. sagittal
    b. coronal   d. oblique

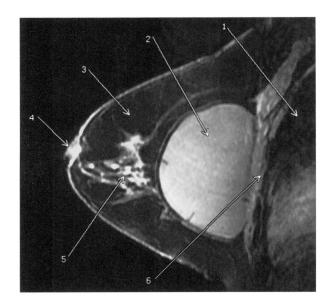

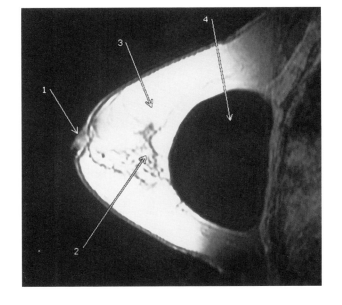

Worksheet 59

Abdomen

Questions 1 to 10 refer to the following figure.

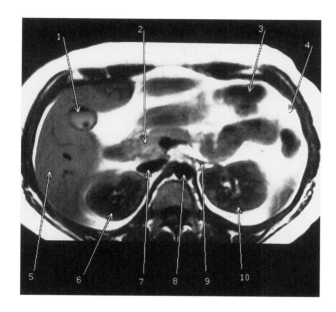

1. Which arrow points to the adrenal gland? _____

2. Which arrow points to the aorta? _____

3. Which arrow points to the bowel? _____

4. Which arrow points to the gallbladder? _____

5. Which arrow points to the inferior vena cava? _____

6. Which arrow points to the left kidney? _____

7. Which arrow points to the liver? _____

8. Which arrow points to the mesentary? _____

9. Which arrow points to the pancreas? _____

10. Which arrow points to the right kidney? _____

Questions 11 to 19 refer to the figure below.

11. Which arrow points to the aorta? _____

12. Which arrow points to the diaphragm? _____

13. Which arrow points to the falciform ligament? _____

14. Which arrow points to the inferior vena cava? _____

15. Which arrow points to the liver? _____

16. Which arrrow points to the omentum? _____

17. Which arrow points to the pancreas? _____

18. Which arrow points to the spleen? _____

19. Which arrow points to the stomach? _____

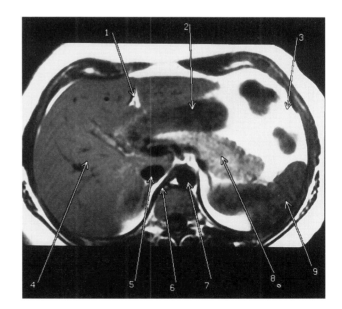

Questions 20 to 31 refer to the figure below.

20. What type of contrast is dominant in this coronal image?

    a. gradient echo T2
    b. inversion recovery T1
    c. spin echo T1
    d. spin echo T2

21. Which arrow points to the abdominal aorta? _____

22. Which arrow points to the adrenal gland? _____

23. Which arrow points to the bowel? _____

24. Which arrow points to the diaphragm? _____

25. Which arrow points to the kidney? _____

26. Which arrow points to the liver? _____

27. Which arrow points to the lung? _____

28. Which arrow points to the mesentary? _____

29. Which arrow points to the psoas muscle? _____

30. Which arrow points to the spleen? _____

31. Which arrow points to the vertebral body? _____

Questions 32 to 34 refer to all of the preceding figures.

32. What type of contrast is dominant in these transverse images of the abdomen?

    a. spin density   c. T2
    b. T1   d. T2*

33. In order to improve contrast resolution in these transverse images a fat suppression technique:

    a. was not necessary b. was used

34. The aorta and the inferior vena cava on both of these transverse images exhibit:

    a. flow voids   b. flow enhancement

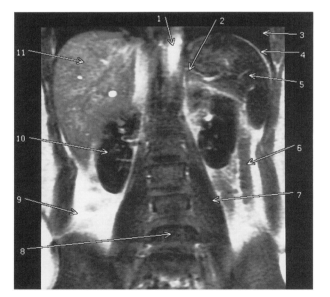

Worksheet 60

Pelvis—Female

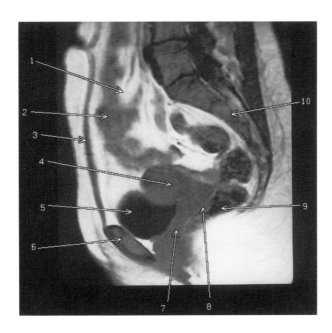

Questions 1 to 11 refer to the figure above.

1. The structures demonstrated in this image are in what anatomical plane?

    a. transverse   c. sagittal
    b. coronal   d. oblique

2. Which arrow points to the bladder? _____

3. Which arrow points to the bowel? _____

4. Which arrow points to the cervix? _____

5. Which arrow points to the mesentary? _____

6. Which arrow points to the pubic bone? _____

7. Which arrow points to the rectum? _____

8. Which arrow points to the rectus abdominus muscle? _____

9. Which arrow points to the sacrum? _____

10. Which arrow points to the uterus? _____

11. Which arrow points to the vagina? _____

12. The structures demonstrated in this image are in what anatomical plane?

    a. transverse   c. sagittal
    b. coronal   d. oblique

13. Which arrow points to the bladder? _____

14. Which arrow points to the external obturator muscle? _____

15. Which arrow points to the internal obturator muscle? _____

16. Which arrow points to the labia? _____

17. Which arrow points to the left ovary? _____

18. Which arrow points to the psoas muscle? _____

19. Which arrow points to the right ovary? _____

20. Which arrow points to the sigmoid colon? _____

21. Which arrow points to the uterus? _____

22. Which arrow points to the vagina? _____

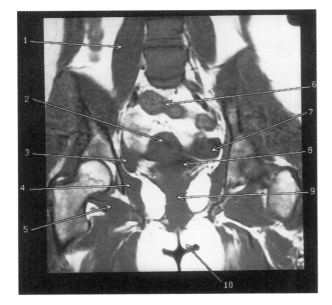

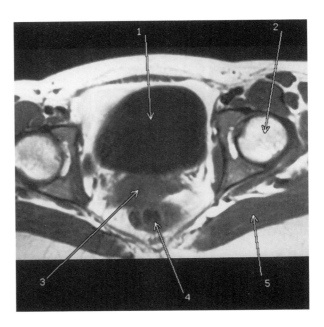

23. The structures demonstrated in this image are in what anatomical plane?

    a. transverse   c. sagittal
    b. coronal   d. oblique

24. Which arrow points to the bladder? _____

25. Which arrow points to the femoral head? _____

26. Which arrow points to the gluteus maximus muscle? _____

27. Which arrow points to the rectum? _____

28. Which arrow points to the vagina? _____

29. What type of contrast is dominant in all of the preceding images of the female pelvis?

    a. spin density   c. T2
    b. T1   d. T2*

Pelvis—Male

Questions 1 to 8 refer to the following figure.

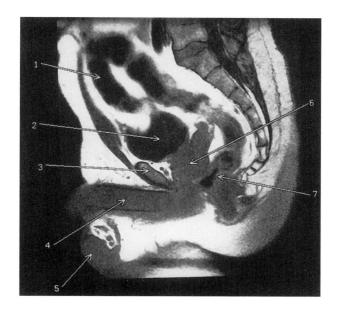

Questions 9 to 14 refer to following figure.

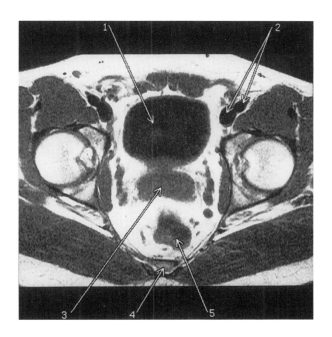

1. What type of contrast is dominant in this image?

   a. spin density   c. T2
   b. T1   d. T2*

2. Which arrow points to the bladder? _____

3. Which arrow points to the bowel? _____

4. Which arrow points to the penis? _____

5. Which arrow points to the prostate gland? _____

6. Which arrow points to the pubic bone? _____

7. Which arrow points to the rectum? _____

8. Which arrow points to the testis? _____

9. What type of contrast is dominant in this image?

   a. spin density   c. T2
   b. T1   d. T2*

10. Which arrow points to the bladder? _____

11. Which arrow points to the femoral vessels? _____

12. Which arrow points to the prostate gland? _____

13. Which arrow points to the rectum? _____

14. Which arrow points to the sacrum? _____

Worksheet | 62

TMJ

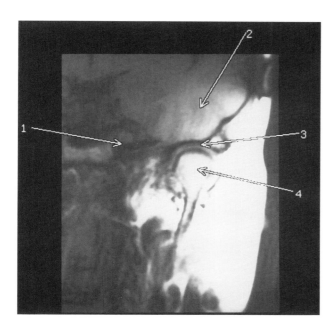

1. When positioning a surface coil for TMJ imaging, the coil should be positioned with its center slightly _____ to the external auditory canal.

   a. anterior   c. posterior
   b. inferior   d. superior

Questions 2 to 6 refer to the above figure.

2. The structures demonstrated in this image are in what anatomical plane?

   a. transverse   c. sagittal
   b. coronal   d. oblique

3. Arrow #1 points to the:

   a. auditory nerve
   b. internal auditory canal
   c. internal carotid artery
   d. middle cerebral artery

4. Arrow #2 points to the:

   a. frontal lobe   c. parietal lobe
   b. occipital lobe   d. temporal lobe

5. Arrow #3 points to the: _____

6. Arrow #4 points to the: _____

Questions 7 to 12 refer to the figure below.

7. The structures demonstrated in this image are in what anatomical plane?

   a. transverse   c. sagittal
   b. coronal   d. oblique

8. Which arrow points to the auditory canal? _____

9. Which arrow points to the intraarticular disc? _____

10. Which arrow points to the mandibular condyle? _____

11. Which arrow points to the mastoid air cells? _____

12. Which arrow points to the temporal lobe? _____

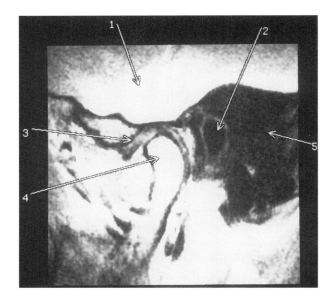

Questions 13 to 20 refer to the following figure.

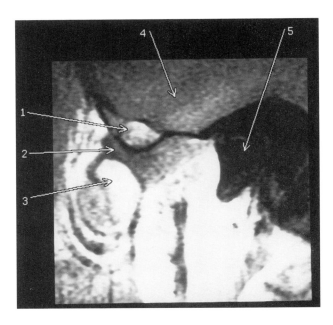

13. The structures demonstrated in this image are in what anatomical plane?

   a. transverse   c. sagittal
   b. coronal   d. oblique

14. Which arrow points to the auditory canal? _____

15. Which arrow points to the intraarticular disc? _____

16. Which arrow points to the mandibular condyle? _____

17. Which arrow points to the temporal bone? _____

18. Which arrow points to the temporal lobe? _____

19. Which of the three images above demonstrates the anatomy in the open-mouth position?

   a. the first image
   b. the second image
   c. the third image

20. In the closed-mouth position, the disk lies with its _____ at the apex of the condyle.

   a. anterior band   c. posterior band
   b. intermediate zone d. superior band

Worksheet 63

Shoulder

Questions 1 to 8 refer to the following figure.

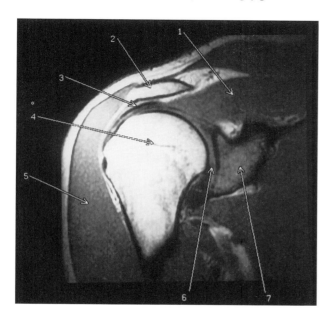

1. The structures demonstrated in this image are in what anatomical plane?

   a. transverse   c. sagittal
   b. coronal   d. oblique

2. Which arrow points to the acromion? _____

3. Which arrow points to the deltoid muscle? _____

4. Which arrow points to the glenoid fossa? _____

5. Which arrow points to the humeral head? _____

6. Which arrow points to the scapula? _____

7. Which arrow points to the spraspinatus muscle? _____

8. Which arrow points to the supraspinatus tendon? _____

Questions 9 to 13 refer to the figure below.

9. The structures demonstrated in this image are in what anatomical plane?

   a. transverse   c. sagittal
   b. coronal   d. oblique

10. Which arrow points to the acromion? _____

11. Which arrow points to the humerus? _____

12. Which arrow points to the rotator cuff? _____

13. What muscle is identified by arrow #4?

    _____

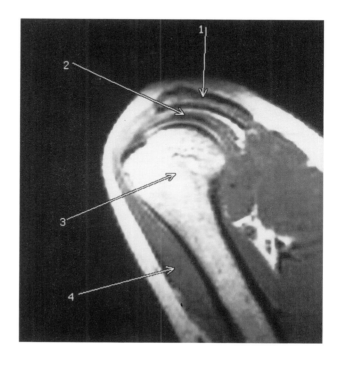

Questions 14 to 25 refer to the two figures below.

14. The structures demonstrated in these images are in what anatomical plane?

    a. transverse   c. sagittal
    b. coronal   d. oblique

15. Which of these two images is the most superior slice?

    a. the first image   b. the second image

16. In the first figure below, which arrow points to the coracoid process? _____

17. In the first figure below, which arrow points to the glenohumeral joint? _____

18. In the first figure below, which arrow points to the humeral head? _____

19. In the first figure below, which arrow points to the scapular spine? _____

20. In the second figure below, which arrow points to the articular cartilage? _____

21. In the second figure below, which arrow points to the deltoid muscle? _____

22. In the second figure below, which arrow points to the humerus? _____

23. In the second figure below, which arrow points to the scapula? _____

24. In the second figure below, which arrow points to the subscapularis tendon? _____

25. What four muscle tendons form the rotator cuff?

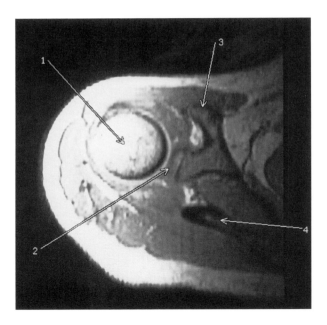

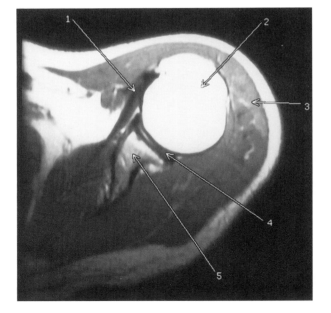

Worksheet 64

Elbow

Questions 1 to 6 refer to the figure below.

1. The structures demonstrated in this image are in what anatomical plane?

   a. transverse   c. sagittal
   b. coronal   d. oblique

2. Which arrow points to the coranoid process? _____

3. Which arrow points to the humerus? _____

4. Which arrow points to the olecranon fossa? _____

5. Which arrow points to the radius? _____

6. Which arrow points to the trochlea? _____

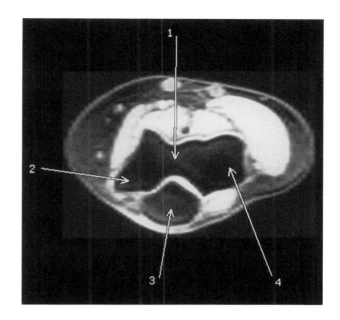

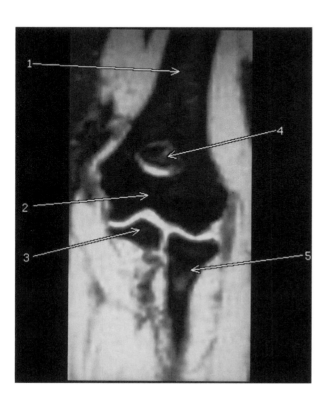

Questions 7 to 11 refer to the figure above.

7. The structures demonstrated in this image are in what anatomical plane?

   a. transverse   c. sagittal
   b. coronal   d. oblique

8. Which arrow points to the lateral epicondyle? _____

9. Which arrow points to the medial epicondyle? _____

10. Which arrow points to the olecranon? _____

11. Which arrow points to the trochlea? _____

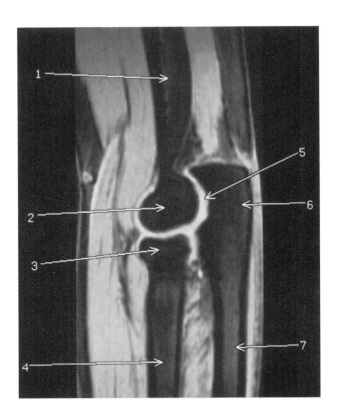

Questions 12 to 19 refer to the figure above.

12. The structures demonstrated in this image are in what anatomical plane?

    a. transverse   c. sagittal
    b. coronal   d. oblique

13. Which arrow points to the humerus? _____

14. Which arrow points to the olecranon? _____

15. Which arrow points to the radial head? _____

16. What arrow points to the radius? _____

17. Which arrow points to the semilunar notch? _____

18. Which arrow points to the trochlea? _____

19. Which arrow points to the ulna? _____

20. In which of the above images was a fat suppression technique used?

    a. all three of the above images
    b. the first and second images
    c. the second and third images
    d. the first and third images

Worksheet | 65

Wrist

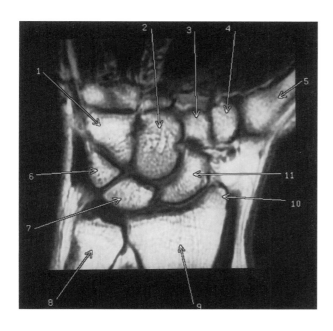

Questions 1 to 12 refer to the above figure.

1. The structures demonstrated in this image are in what anatomical plane?

    a. transverse   c. sagittal
    b. coronal   d. oblique

2. Which arrow points to the capitate? _____

3. Which arrow points to the hamate? _____

4. Which arrow points to the lunate? _____

5. Which arrow points to the metacarpal? _____

6. Which arrow points to the navicular? _____

7. Which arrow points to the radius? _____

8. Which arrow points to the styloid? _____

9. Which arrow points to the trapezium? _____

10. Which arrow points to the trapezoid? _____

11. Which arrow points to the triquetrum? _____

12. Which arrow points to the ulna? _____

Questions 13 to 17 refer to the figure below.

13. The structures demonstrated in this image are in what anatomical plane?

    a. transverse   c. sagittal
    b. coronal   d. oblique

14. Which arrow points to the navicular? _____

15. Which arrow points to the pisiform? _____

16. Which arrow points to the trapezium? _____

17. The #2 arrows are pointing to which group of tendons?

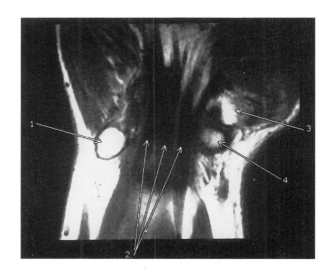

Questions 18 to 22 refer to the following figure.

Questions 23 to 27 refer to the following figure.

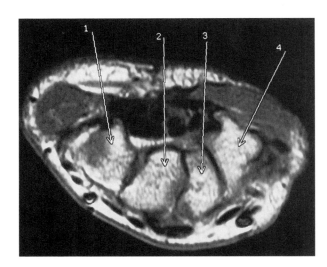

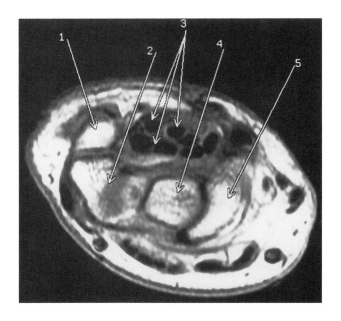

18. The structures demonstrated in this image are in what anatomical plane?

    a. transverse   c. sagittal
    b. coronal   d. oblique

19. Which arrow points to the capitate? _____

20. Which arrow points to the hamate? _____

21. Which arrow points to the trapezium? _____

22. What arrow points to the trapezoid? _____

23. Which arrow points to the flexor tendons? _____

24. Which arrow points to the lunate? _____

25. Which arrow points to the navicular? _____

26. Which arrow points to the pisiform? _____

27. Which arrrow points to the triquetrum? _____

Questions 28 to 32 refer to the figure below.

28. The structures demonstrated in this image are in what anatomical plane?

    a. transverse   c. sagittal
    b. coronal   d. oblique

29. Which arrow points to the capitate? _____

30. Which arrow points to the lunate? _____

31. Which arrow points to the metacarpal? _____

32. What arrow points to the radius? _____

33. Of the two images on page 193, which is the most posterior?

    a. the first image   b. the second image

34. Of the two images on page 194, which is most proximal?

    a. the first image   b. the second image

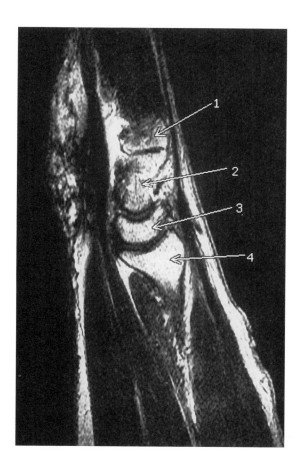

Worksheet | 66

Hips

Questions 1 to 12 refer to the following figure.

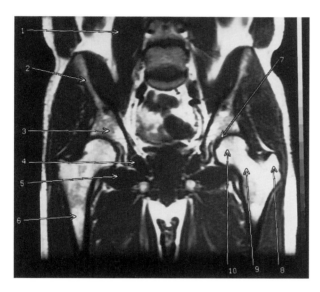

1. What type of contrast is dominant in this image?

   a. spin density   c. T2
   b. T1   d. T2*

2. The structures demonstrated in this image are in what anatomical plane?

   a. transverse   c. sagittal
   b. coronal   d. oblique

3. Which arrow points to the acetabulum? _____

4. Which arrow points to the articular cartilage? _____

5. Which arrow points to the femoral head? _____

6. Which arrow points to the femoral neck? _____

7. Which arrow points to the femur? _____

8. Which arrow points to the greater trochanter? _____

9. Which arrow points to the ilium? _____

10. Which arrow points to the obturator externus? _____

11. Which arrow points to the obturator internus? _____

12. Which arrow points to the psoas muscle? _____

171

Questions 13 to 22 refer to the figure below.

13. The structures demonstrated in this image are in what anatomical plane?

    a. transverse   c. sagittal
    b. coronal   d. oblique

14. Which arrow points to the fat pad? _____

15. Which arrow points to the femoral head? _____

16. Which arrow points to the femoral neck? _____

17. Which arrow points to the gluteus maximus? _____

18. Which arrow points to the ischial tuberosity? _____

19. Which arrow points to the obturator internus?

    _____

20. Which arrow points to the pubic bone? _____

21. Which arrow points to the rectum? _____

22. Which arrow points to the symphysis pubis? _____

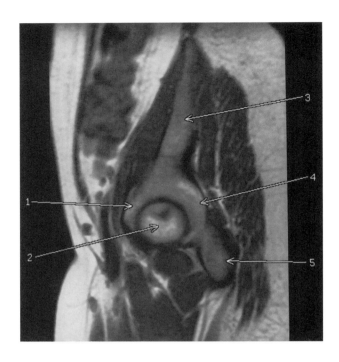

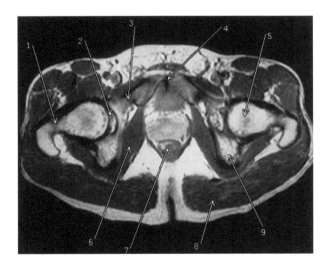

Questions 23 to 28 refer to the above figure.

23. The structures demonstrated in this image are in what anatomical plane?

    a. transverse   c. sagittal
    b. coronal   d. oblique

24. Which arrow points to the femoral head? _____

25. Which arrow points to the ilium? _____

26. Which arrow points to the ischial tuberosity? _____

27. Which arrow points to the ischium? _____

28. Which arrow points to the pubic bone? _____

Worksheet | 67

Knee

Questions 1 to 7 refer to the following figure.

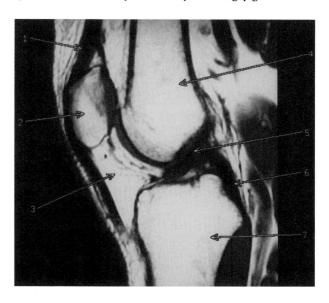

Questions 8 to 12 refer to the following figure.

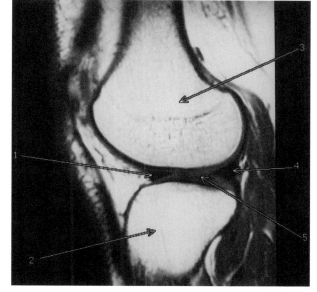

1. Which arrow points to the anterior cruciate ligament? _____

2. Which arrow points to the femur? _____

3. Which arrow points to the infrapatellar fat? _____

4. Which arrow points to the patella? _____

5. Which arrow points to the posterior cruciate ligament? _____

6. Which arrrow points to the quadriceps tendon? _____

7. Which arrow points to the tibia? _____

8. Which arrow points to the anterior lateral meniscus? _____

9. Which arrow points to the articular cartilage? _____

10. Which arrow points to the femur? _____

11. Which arrow points to the posterior lateral meniscus? _____

12. Which arrow points to the tibia? _____

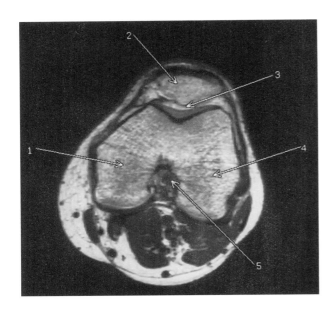

Questions 13 to 17 refer to the figure above.

13. Which arrow points to the anterior cruciate ligament? _____

14. Which arrow points to the lateral condyle? _____

15. Which arrow points to the medial condyle? _____

16. Which arrow points to the patella? _____

17. Which arrow points to the patellar fat? _____

Questions 18 to 26 refer to the figure below.

18. Which arrow points to the anterior cruciate ligament? _____

19. Which arrow points to the lateral condyle? _____

20. Which arrow points to the lateral meniscus? _____

21. Which arrow points to the medial collateral ligament? _____

22. Which arrow points to the medial condyle? _____

23. Which arrow points to the medial meniscus? _____

24. Which arrow points to the posterior cruciate ligament? _____

25. Which arrow points to the tibia? _____

26. Which arrow points to the tibial spine? _____

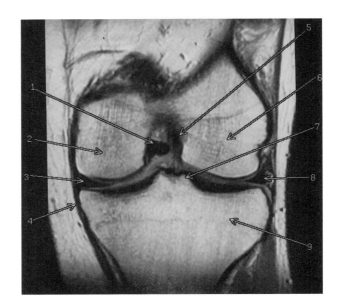

Worksheet | 68

Ankle/Foot

Questions 1 to 10 refer to the following figure.

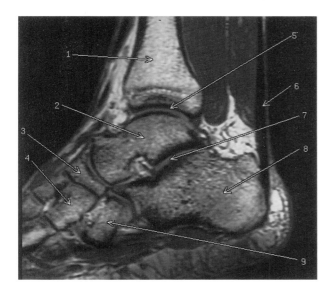

1. The structures demonstrated in this image are in what anatomical plane?

   a. transverse   c. sagittal
   b. coronal   d. oblique

2. Which arrow points to the Achilles tendon? _____

3. Which arrow points to the calcaneous? _____

4. Which arrow points to the cuboid? _____

5. Which arrow points to the lateral cuneiform? _____

6. Which arrow points to the navicular? _____

7. Which arrow points to the subtalar joint? _____

8. Which arrow points to the talus? _____

9. Which arrow points to the tibia? _____

10. Which arrow points to the tibiotalar joint? _____

Questions 11 to 17 refer to the figure below.

11. The structures demonstrated in this image are in what anatomical plane?

    a. transverse   c. sagittal
    b. coronal   d. oblique

12. Which arrow points to the calcaneous? _____

13. Which arrow points to the lateral malleolus? _____

14. Which arrow points to the medial malleolus? _____

15. Which arrow points to the subtalar joint? _____

16. Which arrow points to the talus? _____

17. Which arrow points to the tibia? _____

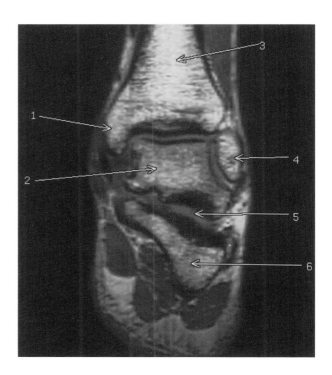

Questions 18 to 22 refer to the following figure.

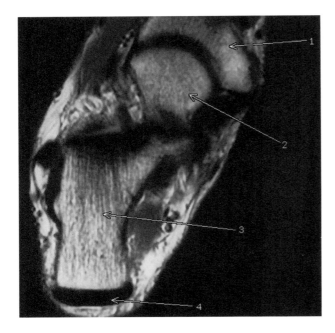

Questions 23 to 32 refer to the following figure.

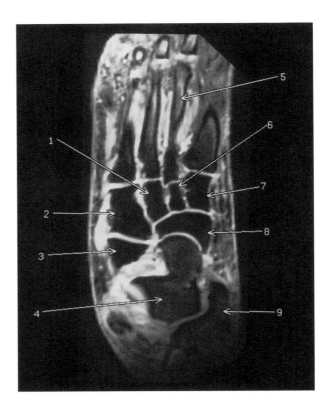

18. The structures demonstrated in this image are in what anatomical plane?

    a. transverse   c. sagittal
    b. coronal   d. oblique

19. Arrow #1 points to the _____

20. Arrow #2 points to the _____

21. Arrow #3 points to the _____

22. Arrow #4 points to the _____

23. The structures demonstrated in this image are in what anatomical plane?

    a. transverse   c. sagittal
    b. coronal   d. oblique

24. Which arrow points to the calcaneous? _____

25. Which arrow points to the cuboid? _____

26. Which arrow points to the intermediate cuneiform? _____

27. Which arrow points to the lateral cuneiform? _____

28. Which arrow points to the medial cuneiform? _____

29. Which arrow points to the medial malleolus? _____

30. Which arrow points to the metatarsal? _____

31. Which arrow points to the navicular? _____

32. Which arrow points to the talus? _____

SECTION IV

Patient Care and MRI Safety

Worksheet | 69 |

Contrast Agents

1. When use of an MR contrast agent causes tissue to appear brighter, _____ has occurred.

   a. spin density contrast
   b. relaxation contrast
   c. positive contrast
   d. negative contrast

2. The use of mineral oil to image the GI tract is an example of enhancing:

   a. electron density
   b. spin density
   c. T1 relaxation
   d. T2 relaxation

3. Ferromagnetic MR contrast agents have the principal characteristic of:

   a. high electron density
   b. high atomic number
   c. high magnetic susceptibility
   d. high spin density

4. Paramagnetic contrast agents are most effective with _____ -weighted pulse sequences.

   a. T1   c. spin density
   b. T2   d. electron density

5. When use of an MR contrast agent results in tissue appearing darker, _____ has occurred.

   a. spin density contrast
   b. relaxation contrast
   c. positive contrast
   d. negative contrast

6. Paramagnetic MRI contrast agents are most commonly based on:
   (1) gadolinium
   (2) dysprosium
   (3) manganese
   (4) iron

   a. 1, 2, and 3   c. 2 and 4
   b. 1 and 3   d. 4 correct

7. Relaxation centers are regions of:

   a. increased spin density
   b. increased magnetization
   c. reduced T1 relaxation
   d. reduced T2 relaxation

8. MR contrast agents are helpful:
   (1) because without them contrast resolution is poor
   (2) by improving disease specificity
   (3) by reducing examination time
   (4) by delineating pathologic processes

   a. 1, 2, and 3   c. 2 and 4
   b. 1 and 3   d. 4

9. One classification of MR contrast agents is according to:

   a. route of administration
   b. mass density
   c. spin density
   d. pulse sequence

10. The use of a paramagnetic agent works by changing:

    a. electron density   c. T1 relaxation times
    b. spin density   d. T2 relaxation times

11. MR contrast agents are:

    a. visualized as increased electron density
    b. visualized as increased spin density
    c. visualized as longer relaxation times
    d. not visualized

12. Contrast agents are helpful in MRI in order to:
    (1) identify regions of decreased tissue profusion
    (2) evaluate blood flow
    (3) image tumors
    (4) identify bony deformities

    a. 1, 2, and 3   c. 2 and 4
    b. 1 and 3   d. 4

13. When classifying MRI contrast agents by route of administration, the possible methods are via:
    (1) ingestion
    (2) inhalation
    (3) IV injection
    (4) IA injection

    a. 1, 2, and 3 c. 2 and 4
    b. 1 and 3   d. all are correct

14. The principle ferromagnetic MR contrast agent is based on:

    a. gadolinium c. iodine
    b. iron oxide   d. water

15. MRI contrast agents principally work through a reduction in:

    a. spin density c. relaxation times
    b. electron density d. flow phenomena

16. An MR contrast agent should:
    (1) alter contrast at low concentrations
    (2) be dose dependent
    (3) be non-toxic
    (4) clear from the body rapidly

    a. 1, 2, and 3 c. 2 and 4
    b. 1 and 3   d. all are correct

17. The use of water loading the kidneys and bladder produces contrast enhancement by changes in:

    a. electron density c. T1 relaxation time
    b. spin density d. T2 relaxation time

18. Paramagnetism is due to:

    a. high atomic number
    b. varying electron density
    c. unpaired orbital electrons
    d. odd numbers of nucleons

19. In general, low concentrations of an MRI contrast agent:

    a. affect T1 more than T2
    b. affect T2 more than T1
    c. affect spin density more than electron density
    d. affect electron density more than spin density

20. MR contrast agents act principally through changing:

    a. mass density c. electron density
    b. spin density d. relaxation times

21. When used with T1-weighted pulse sequences, MRI contrast agents usually result in _____ contrast enhancement.

    a. positive c. no
    b. negative d. variable

22. A chelating agent is one which:

    a. changes spin density
    b. binds with another substance
    c. changes T1 relaxation time
    d. changes T2 relaxation time

23. In most clinical applications paramagnetic contrast agents are used with _____ -weighted images, resulting in _____ contrast enhancement.

    a. T1, positive c. T2, positive
    b. T1, negative d. T2, negative

24. Paramagnetic contrast agents administered intravenously:

    a. increase in effect with time after administration
    b. generally produce negative contrast
    c. are eliminated from normal tissue faster than pathology
    d. work principally by changing spin density

25. In general, ferromagnetic contrast agents:

    a. affect T1 relaxation more than T2 relaxation
    b. affect T2 relaxation more than T1 relaxation
    c. affect spin density more than electron density
    d. affect electron density more than spin density

26. When using paramagnetic contrast agents to produce positive contrast, the effect is due to:

    a. shortening of T1 relaxation time
    b. lengthening of T1 relaxation time
    c. shortening of T2 relaxation time
    d. lengthening of T2 relaxation time

27. Paramagnetic contrast agents administered intravenously are effective for imaging tumors principally because they:

    a. produce positive contrast enhancement
    b. produce negative contrast enhancement
    c. increase spin density
    d. decrease spin density

28. Use of the chelating agent DTPA is effective because it:
    (1) increases spin density
    (2) lowers toxicity
    (3) changes relaxation time
    (4) increases elimination

    a. 1, 2, and 3 c. 2 and 4
    b. 1 and 3   d. 4

29. Ferromagnetic contrast agents when used with T2-weighted pulse sequences produce _____ contrast enhancement.

    a. positive c. no
    b. negative d. variable

30. The commerically available paramagnetic contrast agents are:
    (1) administered only intravenously
    (2) distributed into blood and extracellular space
    (3) nonspecific agents
    (4) organ specific agents

    a. 1, 2, and 3 c. 2 and 4
    b. 1 and 3   d. 4

31. When used as MRI contrast agents, kaolin and bentonite:
    (1) are administered intravenously
    (2) are administered orally
    (3) lengthen T1 relaxation time
    (4) shorten T2 relaxation time

    a. 1, 2, and 3 c. 2 and 4
    b. 1 and 3   d. 4

32. Paramagnetic contrast agents enhance brain tumors by:

    a. changing spin density
    b. crossing the blood-brain barrier
    c. increasing T1 relaxation time
    d. increasing T2 relaxation time

33. Currently the following MRI contrast agents are clinically approved:
    (1) gadolinic acid
    (2) gadoterate meglumine
    (3) gadolinium oxybromide
    (4) gadodiamide

    a. 1, 2, and 3 c. 2 and 4
    b. 1 and 3   d. 4

34. The paramagnetic contrast agents generally:

    a. decrease T1 and increase T2 relaxation times
    b. increase T1 and decrease T2 relaxation times
    c. increase both T1 and T2 relaxation times
    d. decrease both T1 and T2

35. When used as MRI contrast agents, kaolin and bentonite result in negative contrast enhancement on:

    a. both T1- and T2-weighted images
    b. only T1-weighted images
    c. only T2-weighted images
    d. only spin density–weighted images

36. The common characteristic of current MRI contrast agents is:

    a. equal spin density
    b. equal electron density
    c. the metal ion gadolinium
    d. they alter flow

37. Use of paramagnetic contrast agents causes a (an) _____ in the signal intensity on T1-weighted images and a (an) _____ in signal intensity on T2-weighted images.

    a. increase, increase c. decrease, decrease
    b. increase, decrease d. decrease, increase

38. When used as an MRI contrast agent, ferric ammonium citrate:
    (1) is administered orally
    (2) is a ferromagnetic substance
    (3) decreases relaxation times
    (4) increases spin density

    a. 1, 2, and 3 c. 2 and 4
    b. 1 and 3   d. 4

39. Which of the following MRI contrast agents is normally administered via ingestion?

    a. ferric ammonium citrate
    b. oxygen
    c. stable free radicals
    d. hydrogen

40. Which of the following MRI contrast agents is normally administered via IV injection?

    a. barium   c. clay minerals
    b. oxygen   d. gadolinium DTPA

41. What is DTPA?

42. Why is gadolinium such a dynamic contrast media?

43. Name some specific advantages in using Gd-DTPA.

44. What is an unpaired electron?

MRI Energy Fields

1. The suspected biologic effect of the transient magnetic field occurs principally because of:

    a. induced currents   c. polarization
    b. tissue heating   d. relaxation

2. Cultured human cells when exposed to intense static magnetic fields:

    a. grow more slowly
    b. grow more rapidly
    c. die prematurely
    d. show no effect

3. Transient magnetic fields are measured in:

    a. tesla   c. tesla per second
    b. tesla per hertz   d. tesla per cm^2

4. The main potential for a biologic response from RF is:

    a. tissue heating
    b. polarization
    c. induction of currents
    d. suppression of relaxation time

5. Microwave ovens use RF emissions:

    a. of lower frequency than MRI
    b. of higher frequency than MRI
    c. with no electric vector
    d. with no magnetic vector

6. The suspected biologic effect of the RF magnetic field occurs principally because of:

    a. induced currents   c. polarization
    b. tissue heating   d. relaxation

7. Exposing pregnant mice to an intense static magnetic field causes:

    a. growth retardation
    b. congenital abnormalities
    c. malignant disease induction
    d. no effect

8. Electric current density induced by transient magnetic fields is measured in:

    a. tesla per second   c. amperes per second
    b. tesla per cm   d. amperes per cm^2

9. Heating from exposure to an RF field is caused by the:

    a. oscillating electric field
    b. constant electric field
    c. oscillating magnetic field
    d. constant magnetic field

10. Which of the following test subjects, when exposed for a considerable time to the combined fields of MRI, exhibited a biologic response?
    (1) bacteria
    (2) human lymphocytes
    (3) mammalian male chromosomes
    (4) none

    a. 1, 2, and 3   c. 2 and 3
    b. 1 and 3   d. 4

11. The principal responses to a static magnetic field are:
    (1) relaxation
    (2) polarization
    (3) ferromagnetic susceptibility
    (4) ferromagnetic projectiles

    a. 1, 2, and 3   c. 2 and 4
    b. 1 and 3   d. all are correct

12. A transient magnetic field can also be called:
    (1) a moving magnetic field
    (2) an integrated magnetic field
    (3) a time-varying magnetic field
    (4) a differential magnetic field

    a. 1, 2, and 3   c. 2 and 4
    b. 1 and 3   d. all are correct

13. The current density induced by transient magnetic fields depends mainly on:
    (1) repetition time
    (2) tissue conductivity
    (3) spin density
    (4) time of field activation

    a. 1, 2, and 3   c. 2 and 4
    b. 1 and 3   d. all are correct

14. The energy absorbed in a patient from an RF field is a function of:
    (1) frequency
    (2) exposure time
    (3) patient mass
    (4) patient fat content

    a. 1, 2, and 3   c. 2 and 4
    b. 1 and 3   d. all are correct

15. Low frequency electromagnetic fields (EMF) relate to:

    a. typical household electricity
    b. MRI
    c. microwave radiation
    d. ultrasonic diathermy

16. The intensity response relationship that best describes MRI biologic effects is:

    a. linear, nonthreshold
    b. linear, threshold
    c. nonlinear, nonthreshold
    d. nonlinear, threshold

17. When a patient is removed from an MR imager, some tissues of the patient:

    a. remain polarized forever
    b. lose their polarization over time
    c. return to normal immediately
    d. lose their spin density

18. The principal potential effect of a transient magnetic field is to:

    a. alter spin density
    b. alter relaxation time
    c. induce magnetic domains
    d. induce electrical currents

19. Because biologic effects of MRI fields are threshold in nature:

    a. some intensities are absolutely safe
    b. no intensity is absolutely safe
    c. response increases rapidly with intensity
    d. response is level with increasing intensity

20. The earthís magnetic field in the United States is approximately:

    a. 10 microtesla   c. 100 microtesla
    b. 25 microtesla   d. 250 microtesla

21. The following MRI energy fields have the potential to induce a biologic response:
    (1) the RF field
    (2) the acoustic field
    (3) the transient magnetic field
    (4) the geometric field

    a. 1, 2, and 3   c. 2 and 4
    b. 1 and 3   d. all are correct

22. Which of the following studies that exposed rodents to intense static magnetic fields resulted in positive findings?
    (1) growth retardation
    (2) congenital abnormalities
    (3) malignant disease induction
    (4) none

    a. 1, 2, and 3   c. 2 and 3
    b. 1 and 3   d. 4

23. The interaction between transient magnetic fields and tissue is due to:

    a. radiation absorption
    b. electromagnetic induction
    c. electromagnetic radiation
    d. radiation induction

24. The suspected biologic effect of the static magnetic field occurs principally because of:

    a. induced currents   c. polarization
    b. tissue heating   d. relaxation

25. The term orthogonal means:

    a. in the same direction as
    b. around a point
    c. perpendicular to
    d. throughout a volume

26. The radio frequency range employed in MRI covers approximately:

  a. 1 to 10 megahertz
  b. 10 to 100 megahertz
  c. 100 to 1000 megahertz
  d. 1000 to 10,000 megahertz

27. RF energy deposition is expressed as:

  a. specific absorption rate
  b. specific ionization potential
  c. thermal absorption energy
  d. absorption coefficient

28. The earth's magnetic field is:

  a. less than that associated with household appliances
  b. more that that associated with household appliances
  c. about the same as an MRI
  d. about the same as that at the exclusion line of an MRI

29. The units of specific absorption rate (SAR) are:

  a. tesla per second   c. watts per cm²
  b. tesla per hertz   d. watts per kilogram

30. Match the following MRI field descriptions with the possible response.
  (1) induced currents; (2) tissue heating;
  (3) trauma; (4) polarization

  a. static magnetic field   _____
  b. transient magnetic field   _____
  c. RF field   _____
  d. ferromagnetic attraction   _____

31. Which of the lines on the following figure are orthogonal to one another?

  a. A   c. C
  b. B   d. D

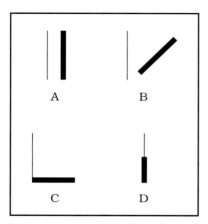

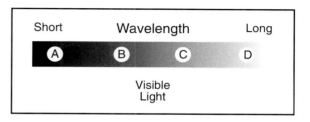

32. Which region in the above rendering of the electromagnetic spectrum is RF?

  a. A   c. C
  b. B   d. D

QUESTIONS TO PONDER

33. Can a permanent magnet MR imager with its relatively low B_0 create ferromagnetic projectiles?

34. In what units is SAR measured?

35. What is the most important factor that could cause an imaging procedure to exceed the FDA SAR guidelines?

Human Responses to MRI

1. Some biologic responses have been reported in subjects imaged with 4 T research imagers. These include:
   (1) metallic taste
   (2) twitching
   (3) disequilibrium
   (4) phosphene induction

   a. 1, 2, and 3   c. 2 and 4
   b. 1 and 3   d. all are correct

2. The threshold for induction of magnetic phosphenes at low frequencies is approximately:

   a. 1 T/s   c. 10 T/s
   b. 3 T/s   d. 30 T/s

3. The current density threshold for ventricular fibrillation is thought to be approximately:

   a. 0.1 mA/cm^2 c. 1 mA/cm^2
   b. 0.5 mA/cm^2 d. 5 mA/cm^2

4. Human responses have been observed following exposure to:
   (1) transient magnetic fields
   (2) static magnetic fields
   (3) RF emissions
   (4) none of the above

   a. 1, 2, and 3   c. 2 and 3
   b. 1 and 3   d. 4

5. The human responses reported during imaging with a 4 T system are presumed to be due to:

   a. the static magnetic field
   b. the transient magnetic field
   c. the radio frequency field
   d. ferromagnetic projectiles

6. The potential hazard to patients from RF irradiation is principally due to:

   a. ionization   c. current induction
   b. excitation   d. tissue heating

7. The highest static magnetic field that can be comfortably tolerated is probably:

   a. 2 T   c. much higher than 4 T
   b. 4 T   d. unbounded

8. Bone healing is helped by:

   a. low frequency RF
   b. high frequency RF
   c. static magnetic fields
   d. transient magnetic fields

9. Magnetic phosphenes:
   (1) are caused by static magnetic fields
   (2) are caused by transient magnetic fields
   (3) result in spin density changes
   (4) result in light flashes

   a. 1, 2, and 3   c. 2 and 4
   b. 1 and 3   d. all are correct

10. The USFDA limits the SAR averaged over the whole body to:

    a. 0.4 W/kg   c. 4 W/kg
    b. 2 W/kg   d. 20 W/kg

11. Probably the most common biologic response of an MRI patient is:

    a. claustrophobia   c. agitation
    b. sleep   d. nerve stimulation

12. The maximum permissible static magnetic field is limited by the USFDA to:

    a. 1 tesla   c. 4 tesla
    b. 2 tesla   d. 8 tesla

13. The USFDA limits the transient magnetic field of a clinical MRI imager to:

    a. 1 T/s   c. 10 T/s
    b. 3 T/s   d. 30 T/s

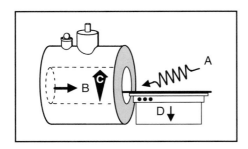

14. Which letter in in the above figure represents the field that can create ferromagnetic projectiles?

    a. A   c. C
    b. B   d. D

◻ **QUESTIONS TO PONDER**

15. Stainless steel is not ferromagnetic. Can it become a projectile?

16. What MRI energy field is associated with thermal energy deposited in tissue?

General Safety Considerations

1. On beginning an MR examination, patient anxiety is generally due to:

   a. drowsiness
   b. claustophobia
   c. irritability
   d. sleeplessness

2. It is recommended that the fringe magnetic field be access controlled to:

   a. 0.1 mT
   b. 0.5 mT
   c. 1 mT
   d. 5 mT

3. The most clinically important hazard from MRI involves:

   a. polarization of the patient
   b. the induction of electric currents
   c. focal heating
   d. ferromagnetic projectiles

4. Claustrophobia is the fear of:

   a. tunnels
   b. heights
   c. confined spaces
   d. large rooms

5. Ferromagnetic surgical clips are hazardous because they:

   a. can be pulled from the patient
   b. may heat up excessively
   c. may twist to align with the static magnetic field
   d. may rotate out of the field of view

6. Studies with the energy fields of MRI and pregnant animals or humans suggest that:

   a. there is no effect
   b. the effect is minimal and transient
   c. the affect is minimal but progressive
   d. malignant disease can be induced

7. Approximately _____ of all patients exhibit some claustrophobia.

   a. 1%
   b. 5%
   c. 20%
   d. 50%

8. How should one determine that surgical clips are not magnetic prior to use?

   a. bring them to the MRI magnet
   b. observe them in the presence of a hand magnet
   c. expose them in a microwave oven
   d. expose them to a magnetic cleaner

9. A helpful technique to get claustrophobics through the examination is to:

   a. have them take a nap first
   b. have them drink lots of water
   c. position a friend in contact with them
   d. let them listen to music

10. Which of the following contraindicate MRI examination:
    (1) cardiac pacemakers
    (2) hemostat clips
    (3) neuro stimulators
    (4) orthopedic implants

    a. 1, 2, and 3
    b. 1 and 3
    c. 2 and 4
    d. all are correct

11. Pacemakers can be interrupted at static magnetic fields of approximately:

    a. 2 mT
    b. 5 mT
    c. 10 mT
    d. 50 mT

12. Earplugs should be used for hearing protection since the gradient switching can produce sound levels up to approximately:

    a. 25 dB
    b. 50 dB
    c. 100 dB
    d. 150 dB

13. Which letter in the following figure represents the field that can elevate body temperature?

    a. A   c. C
    b. B   d. D

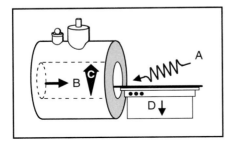

14. What is the relationship of the Kelvin scale to the Celsius scale and the Farenheit scale?

15. Why should MR operators not wear gold earrings when it is known that gold is not ferromagnetic?

16. What measures can be instituted to reduce claustrophobia?

Worksheet 73

Equipment and Human Resources

1. Having decided to establish an MR imaging facility, the first step in such a process is:

   a. select the imager   c. propose a time line
   b. staff the facility   d. identify the location

2. To ensure that potential ferromagnetic projectiles do not enter the imaging room one should use:

   a. a portal sensing device
   b. an airport type surveillance fluoroscope
   c. a dedicated radiographic unit
   d. a small magnet

3. MRI technologists may:
   (1) be trained on the job
   (2) attend vendor-sponsored training programs
   (3) require no training
   (4) have completed acceptable MRI training courses

   a. 1, 2, and 3   c. 2 and 4
   b. 1 and 3   d. 4

4. Continuing education of MR technologists is important so they can exercise independent judgment principally in:

   a. patient positioning
   b. patient preparation
   c. magnetic field strength selection
   d. scan protocol implementation

5. Perhaps the most important part of patient preparation is:

   a. a scheduled date and time
   c. treatment at the reception desk
   b. an interview with the radiologist
   d. preparation by the MRI technologist

6. When preparing the patient for examination, the MR technologist should:
   (1) describe the thumping noises to be heard
   (2) relate the time of the examination
   (3) emphasize the importance of remaining still
   (4) be sure the patient knows this is a diagnostic examination, not a treatment

   a. 1, 2, and 3   c. 2 and 4
   b. 1 and 3   d. all are correct

7. A major consideration for placement of items in the imaging room is

   a. cost   c. magnetic property
   b. convenience   d. staffing requirement

8. Acceptable ferromagnetic items that can be placed in the imaging room are:
   (1) fire extinguishers
   (2) oxygen cylinders
   (3) wheelchairs
   (4) patient monitors

   a. 1, 2, and 3   c. 2 and 4
   b. 1 and 3   d. none are correct

9. Who of the following would be best to train as an MR technologist?
   (1) CT technologists
   (2) radiation therapists
   (3) ultrasonographers
   (4) student technologists

   a. 1, 2, and 3   c. 2 and 4
   b. 1 and 3   d. 4

10. Which of the following are of particular importance in the successful administration of an MR imaging facility?
    (1) patient scheduling
    (2) patient preparation
    (3) technologist skills
    (4) report generation

    a. 1, 2, and 3   c. 2 and 4
    b. 1 and 3   d. all are correct

11. During the MRI examination:
    (1) contact with the patient is necessary
    (2) ferromagnetic materials should be removed
    (3) patient motion should cease
    (4) the technologist may break after setting the scan protocol

    a. 1, 2, and 3   c. 2 and 4
    b. 1 and 3   d. all are correct

12. Which of the following is essential for MRI start-up?
    (1) fire code
    (2) crash cart
    (3) patient stimulator
    (4) magnet detector

    a. 1, 2, and 3   c. 2 and 4
    b. 1 and 3   d. 4

13. Patient sedation for an MRI examination will be necessary approximately once:

    a. a day   c. every other week
    b. a week   d. a month

14. _____ usually results in MR images that appear bright.

    a. lung tissue   c. strong signal intensity
    b. fat tissue   d. rapid pulse sequences

15. Successful MRI operation must include:

    a. sending a postcard to remind each patient of the scheduled examination time
    b. calling each outpatient the day before the scheduled examination
    c. having the patient show up one hour before examination time
    d. requiring the radiologist to interview the patient prior to examination

16. If the presence of foreign ferromagnetic material in the patient is questionable:
    (1) radiographs may be taken
    (2) sonograms may be taken
    (3) CT images may be obtained
    (4) fluoroscopy should be done

    a. 1, 2, and 3   c. 2 and 4
    b. 1 and 3   d. all are correct

17. As operation of an MR imager becomes more routine, in all likelihood:
    (1) less ancillary equipment will be required
    (2) costs will decline
    (3) examination time will decrease
    (4) more ancillary equipment will be required

    a. 1, 2, and 3   c. 2 and 4
    b. 1 and 3   d. 4

18. The cost of establishing an MRI facility is so high that optimum utilization should be:

    a. 8 hours a day, 5 days a week
    b. 12 hours a day, 5 days a week
    c. 18 hours a day, 5 days a week
    d. 18 hours a day, 6 days a week

19. Continuing education and training of MR technologists is:

    a. unnecessary   c. desirable
    b. unimportant   d. essential

20. A consent form for an MRI examination is necessary when:

    a. the imager is brand new
    b. any imager components are not USFDA approved
    c. the imager has been repaired recently
    d. it is the patient's first MRI examination

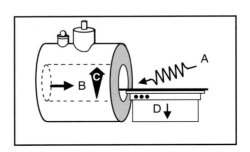

21. Which letter in the figure above represents the field which can induce magnetophosphenes?

    a. A   c. C
    b. B   d. D

☐ **QUESTIONS TO PONDER**

22. How do surgical clips affect image quality?

23. What can the operator do to minimize superficial burns?

24. What is SAR?

25. What effect does a prosthesis have on image quality?

Worksheet 74

Scanning Protocols/Maintenance

1. The primary responsibility of the MR technologist is to:

   a. prepare the patient
   b. image the patient
   c. select the optimum imaging parameters
   d. report the results in a timely fashion

2. Pulse sequences optimized for imaging the CNS are usually not appropriate for body imaging because for CNS compared with body tissues:

   a. T1 and T2 are long
   b. T1 is long and T2 is short
   c. T1 is short and T2 is long
   d. T1 and T2 are short

3. Cryogen levels should be monitored:

   a. hourly   c. weekly
   b. daily   d. monthly

4. Maintenance costs can be controlled if:

   a. patients are not scheduled too frequently
   b. all service engineers are properly trained
   c. repairs are done after hours
   d. preventive maintenance is done after hours

5. Liquid helium has a vaporization temperature of:

   a. 0 K   c. 19 K
   b. 4 K   d. 77 K

6. If a cryogenerator is not a part of the magnet, boil off liquid helium amounts to approximately _____ percent per day.

   a. 1   c. 10
   b. 5   d. 20

7. Should a quench occur and helium escapes, the principle effect on the MR technologist will be:

   a. lowered body temperature
   b. skin rash
   c. superficial burn
   d. Donald Duck voice

8. In general, MR technologists select pulse sequence parameters that will:

   a. reduce motion artifacts
   b. minimize SAR
   c. use least imager time
   d. provide most information in the least time

9. A minimum of _____ hours per month is needed for regular cryogen replacement and preventive maintenance.

   a. three   c. fourteen
   b. seven   d. twenty-four

10. Liquid nitrogen has a vaporization temperature of:

   a. 0 K   c. 20 K
   b. 4 K   d. 77 K

11. If a cryogenerator is not a part of the magnet, boil off liquid nitrogen amounts to approximately _____ percent per day.

   a. 1   c. 20
   b. 5   d. 40

12. Proper quality control for an MR imager requires that phantom studies be performed:

   a. daily   c. biweekly
   b. weekly   d. monthly

193

13. Routinely, double echo imaging is employed to provide:

    a. spin density–weighted images for anatomy and T1-weighted images for pathology
    b. spin density–weighted images for anatomy and T2-weighted images for pathology
    c. T1-weighted images for anatomy and T2-weighted images for pathology
    d. T2-weighted images for anatomy and T1-weighted imaged for pathology

14. In addition to the main magnet the following support systems normally require preventive maintenance:
    (1) the emergency generator
    (2) the air conditioning system
    (3) the oxygen alarm system
    (4) the nonmagnetic video

    a. 1, 2, and 3   c. 2 and 4
    b. 1 and 3   d. all are correct

15. Potentially harmful changes in the RF subsystem result because of:

    a. excessive SAR
    b. amplitude reduction
    c. patient loading
    d. frequency drift

16. Abrupt loss of cryogens results in:

    a. magnet quench
    b. Larmor frequency shift
    c. spin density reduction
    d. relaxation time reduction

17. The principle hazard with handling cryogenic gases is:

    a. freezing   c. irritation
    b. burning   d. rash

18. The critical level of fill of cryogenic gases above which a quench is not likely is approximately:

    a. 10%   c. 50%
    b. 25%   d. 75%

19. Of all of the quality control measurements _____ is perhaps the most important.

    a. artifact generation   c. magnet homogeneity
    b. signal-to-noise   d. distortion

20. During spin echo, imaging increases in _____ signal intensity and increases in _____ signal intensities.

    a. T1 increase, T2 increase
    b. T1 reduce, T2 increase
    c. T1 increase, T2 reduce
    d. T1 reduce, T2 reduce

21. Cryogen replacement is considerably reduced with the installation of a:

    a. halon system   c. magnetometer
    b. cryogenerator   d. hall effect gauss meter

22. The primary element(s) of an MR imager requiring repair and service is:

    a. electronic components
    b. the main magnet
    c. the gradient coils
    d. the halon system

23. The critical temperature for superconductivity is approximately:

    a. 0 K   c. 20 K
    b. 9 K   d. 77 K

24 On those magnets cooled with helium and nitrogen, cryogenic gas replenishment may be required as often as _____ for helium and _____ for nitrogen.

    a. daily, daily   c. weekly, monthly
    b. weekly, weekly   d. monthly, monthly

25 The Charles law of gases states that at constant pressure:

    a. the temperature is proportional to mass density
    b. the temperature is proportional to spin density
    c. the volume is proportional to mass density
    d. the volume is proportional to temperature

26. The only time the main magnet should require service is when:

    a. there is a fire
    b. a quench occurs
    c. spin density changes
    d. one or more frequencies change

27. The critical temperature for superconductivity is approximately:

    a. -250° C   c. -100° C
    b. -150° C   d. 0° C

28. Which of the following is an image characteristic that should be routinely evaluated in a quality assurance program?
    (1) signal-to-noise ratio
    (2) spatial resolution
    (3) contrast resolution
    (4) sensitivity profile

    a. 1, 2, and 3   c. 2 and 4
    b. 1 and 3   d. all are correct

29. Quality control programs recommend a (an) _____ performance evaluation by a qualified medical physicist.

    a. weekly   c. biannual
    b. monthly   d. annual

30. Which letter in the figure below represents room temperature?

    a. A   c. C
    b. B   d. D

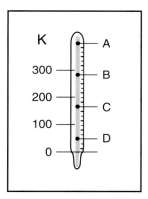

⬛ QUESTIONS TO PONDER

31. Is image quality affected if the pulse sequence is altered for claustrophobic patients?

32. What is the advised precautionary procedure when one questions the magnetic susceptibility of a particular prosthesis?

33. When will dental fillings present imaging problems?

34. Why are both CT and MRI images often obtained on the same patient?

35. How can the operator know if the presaturation slices are correctly applied?

Worksheet 75

Safety

1. Principle hazards to patients and personnel in an MRI facility is the biologic effect of:

   a. the main magnetic field
   b. the transient magnetic field
   c. the RF field
   d. ferromagnetic projectiles

2. Which of the following personal effects should be removed from visitors and patients before entering the MR imaging room?
   (1) credit cards
   (2) calculators
   (3) jewelry
   (4) beepers

   a. 1, 2, and 3   c. 2 and 4
   b. 1 and 3   d. all are correct

3. The following people present as potentially unacceptable patients:
   (1) welders
   (2) beauticians
   (3) auto mechanics
   (4) nurses

   a. 1, 2, and 3   c. 2 and 4
   b. 1 and 3   d. all are correct

4. Patients containing neurosurgical clips and implants may be imaged:

   a. if the surgery was within the last three years
   b. if the surgical report shows the device was nonmagnetic
   c. if the device is shown nonmagnetic following radiography
   d. never

5. Joint prosthesis in a patient may:

   a. be a contraindication for MRI
   b. heat unacceptably, due to RF exposure
   c. be pulled from the patient
   d. degrade the image

6. An absolute requirement of management before opening an MR imaging facility is:
   (1) in-service training of building personnel
   (2) specification of Larmor frequency
   (3) ensuring pacemaker patients do not enter
   (4) provision for nonmagnetic video

   a. 1, 2, and 3   c. 2 and 4
   b. 1 and 3   d. all are correct

7. A clearly marked exclusion area should be identified at the:

   a. 0.1 mT fringe field c. 0.5 mT fringe field
   b. 0.3 mT fringe field d. 1 mT fringe field

8. A patient with a history of intraorbital metal can be imaged if:

   a. the metal is identified radiographically
   b. the metal is identified fluoroscopically
   c. the metal is considered nonmagnetic
   d. never

9. Middle ear prosthetic devices may:

   a. torque, causing injury
   b. be pulled from the patient
   c. rotate at the Larmor frequency
   d. cause image degradation

10. The pregnant patient:

    a. should not be imaged with MRI
    b. should not be imaged in the first trimester with MRI
    c. can be imaged at any time, provided the results will materially affect patient management
    d. can be imaged at any time, following completion of satisfactory consent forms

11. The following items are usually safe to take into the MR imaging room:
    (1) a gold watch
    (2) a semiconductor watch
    (3) credit cards
    (4) a laser pointer

    a. 1, 2, and 3   c. 2 and 4
    b. 1 and 3   d. all are correct

12. The responsiblity of recognizing a potentially unacceptable patient for MR imaging rests with the:

    a. receptionist   c. technologist
    b. nurse   d. radiologist

13. If foreign metallic objects are suspected, _____ is acceptable for identification and exclusion of the patient.
    (1) radiography
    (2) sonography
    (3) CT examination
    (4) fluoroscopy

    a. 1, 2, and 3   c. 2 and 4
    b. 1 and 3   d. all are correct

14. Abdominal surgical clips in a patient may:

    a. be a contraindication for MRI
    b. torque creating vessel rupture
    c. be pulled from the patient
    d. reduce image quality

15. Surgical clips in the brain may contraindicate MRI because of which energy field (refer to the following figure)?

    a. A   c. C
    b. B   d. D

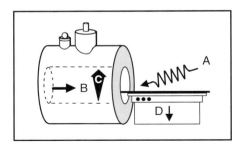

☐ QUESTIONS TO PONDER

16. Who is more susceptible to a claustrophobic response—a male or a female?

17. What precautionary measures should be taken before imaging the head of a patient that has a history as a machinist, lathe operator, etc?

18. What is the USFDA? the USCDRH?

SECTION V

Appendices

Appendix A

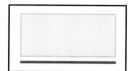

Worksheet Answers

Worksheet Number 1

1. d	10. d	19. a
2. d	11. c	20. d
3. d	12. 1, 4, 2, 3	21. c
4. b	13. c	22. c
5. c	14. b	23. c
6. 3, 2, 4, 1	15. 4, 2, 1, 3	24. 4, 2, 3, 1
7. d	16. 2, 4, 1, 3	
8. c	17. 2, 4, 1, 3	
9. b	18. c	

QTP

25. 5 s = 5000 ms.
26. The electron binding energy in tissue is greater than B_o, B_{xyz} and RF energy fields.
27. Orthogonal refers to the three axes of a vector diagram, each one orthogonal or perpendicular to the other two.
28. X-rays have more energy and shorter wavelength than light. RF has less energy and longer wavelength than light.

Worksheet Number 2

1. b	10. a	19. a
2. a	11. b	20. d
3. a	12. a	21. b
4. d	13. b	22. a
5. b	14. b	23. c
6. d	15. b	24. b
7. c	16. b	25. c
8. c	17. b	
9. c	18. a	

QTP

26. MR has better contrast resolution than both radiography and CT.
27. MR and CT have approximately the same spatial resolution, but radiography is better.
28. Calcium absorbs x-rays and is represented by no atomic silver (white) in the latent image of a radiograph. Calcium produces no MRI signal since its gyromagnetic ratio is different from hydrogen.
29. There are $1000\mu m/mm$, $10,000\mu m/cm$, and $1,000,000\mu m/m$.

Worksheet Number 3

1.	c	10.	a	19.	4, 3, 2,1	28.	d	37. d
2.	c	11.	b	20.	d	29.	b	
3.	a	12.	a	21.	b	30.	d	
4.	d	13.	d	22.	d	31.	a	
5.	c	14.	b	23.	c	32.	b	
6.	c	15.	a	24.	a	33.	a	
7.	d	16.	a	25.	a	34.	b	
8.	c	17.	c	26.	c	35.	b	
9.	b	18.	d	27.	c	36.	a	

QTP

38. The net magnetization is zero because the proton dipole spins are randomly directed.
39. There are no moving parts in an MR imager.
40. M_{xy} is the intensity of net magnetization in the XY plane. It is due to the phase coherence of spins.

Worksheet Number 4

1.	d	10.	d	19.	a	28. c	
2.	b	11.	c	20.	c		
3.	b	12.	d	21.	b		
4.	d	13.	c	22.	c		
5.	c	14.	a	23.	b		
6.	d	15.	c	24.	c		
7.	c	16.	c	25.	c		
8.	a	17.	d	26.	d		
9.	b	18.	a	27.	c		

QTP

29. Static electricity is created by resting electrical charges and is measured in coulombs. Excess electrons on a surface or object are static electricity.
30. These lines would radiate out from each charge but be deflected from each other halfway between the electrons.
31. Emf is electric potential, and it is measured in volts.

Worksheet Number 5

1.	c	10.	d	19.	3, 1, 4, 2
2.	d	11.	c		
3.	a	12.	3, 4, 2, 1		
4.	a	13.	3, 1, 4, 3		
5.	d	14.	c		
6.	a	15.	c		
7.	b	16.	b		
8.	a	17.	b		
9.	c	18.	d		

QTP

20. Electricity is the flow of electrons In a conductor, such as copper. It is measured in amperes.
21. Ohms law describes the relationship between electrical potential, volts (V), electric current (I) and resistance (R). V = IR
22. A conductor is any material allowing the flow of electrons. An insulator will inhibit the flow of electrons.
23. A watt is the unit of electric power. It is the product of volts and amps. 1 W = 1 V x 1 A.

Worksheet Number 6

1. d	10. a	19. 4, 3, 1, 2
2. d	11. d	20. d
3. d	12. b	21. c
4. c	13. d	22. c
5. b	14. d	23. d
6. a	15. b	24. a
7. c	16. b	25. a
8. d	17. c	
9. d	18. d	

QTP

26. The earth's magnetic field measures approximately 100 μT at both poles and 25 μT at the equator.
27. By convention, the magnetic field generated by the north pole will seek the south pole and form one continuous magnetic field that exits the north pole and enters the south pole. In a plane through the imaginary equator the strength of the magnetic field decreases inversely as the square of the distance from the axis.
28. The greater the number of unpaired electrons in an element, the greater will be its magnetic properties.
29. 10,000 G = 1 T
        10 G = 1 mT
         5 G = 0.5 mT
30. Place iron filings on cardboard which rests on a magnet. The iron filings become oriented with the imaginary magnetic field lines.

Worksheet Number 7

1. c	10. c	19. b
2. c	11. b	20. 2, 1, 4, 3
3. d	12. a	
4. c	13. d	
5. d	14. c	
6. c	15. b	
7. c	16. d	
8. c	17. d	
9. d	18. b	

QTP

21. A helix, also called a spiral, is the geometric shape of a coil. A solenoid is a wire helix that conducts electricity.
22. Eddy currents are secondary reverse electric currents induced by magnetic fields in gradient coils that interfere with their operation.

Worksheet Number 8

1. a	10. b	19. b	28. b
2. c	11. d	20. a	29. b
3. c	12. c	21. b	30. c
4. c	13. d	22. b	31. c
5. d	14. a	23. d	32. a
6. c	15. b	24. 2, 4, 3, 1	33. b
7. c	16. b	25. a	34. d
8. d	17. a	26. d	35. c
9. c	18. d	27. b	36. a

QTP

37. The left superscript represents the atomic mass number (A) or the number of protons plus neutrons, and the left subscript the atomic number (Z) or the number of protons.
38. Covalent-bonded molecules share their outer electrons in the bonding process. In ionic bonding the electrons are actually given up from one atom to another.

1. c	10. b	19. d	28. a	37. c
2. d	11. a	20. b	29. a	38. b
3. d	12. d	21. d	30. a	39. d
4. a	13. a	22. a	31. a	40. c
5. a	14. b	23. d	32. d	41. d
6. b	15. c	24. a	33. c	42. c
7. d	16. b	25. b	34. b	43. c
8. c	17. c	26. b	35. d	44. a
9. a	18. c	27. c	36. d	45. b

QTP

46. Cryogenic gases are required to maintain the niobium/titanium superconducting wire at a lower than critical temperature in a zero resistance state.
47. The electric current is reversed, causing the magnetic field to reverse. Gradient reversal can create a gradient echo in GE imaging.
48. The computer reconstructs the image from the digitized signal detected by the RF probe.
49. All systems possess inherent magnetic inhomogeneities because the shimming process is not absolute, but good to only a few parts per million.
50. The RF coils are closest to the patient. The gradient coils are next.

Worksheet Number 10

1. c	10. b	19. a
2. b	11. b	20. c
3. c	12. d	21. b
4. b	13. c	22. d
5. b	14. b	23. a
6. b	15. a	
7. c	16. a	
8. a	17. a	
9. d	18. a	

QTP

24. The B_o field of a permanent magnet is always on. It only requires a matter of minutes to energize a resistive magnet. A superconducting electromagnet imager may require up to an hour if it has been moved or reinstalled.
25. Permanent magnet systems require little electrical power and no cooling. They also have a very low fringe magnetic field.
26. There are three types of MR magnets: permanent magnets, resistive electromagnets and superconductive electromagnets.
27. A quench is caused when the cryostat loses sufficient liquid helium to cause the B_o conductor to change from the superconducting state to the resistive state. More heat is generated and more liquid helium vaporized.

Worksheet Number 11

1. a	10. d	19. b
2. a	11. d	20. d
3. d	12. a	21. d
4. c	13. c	
5. d	14. d	
6. b	15. b	
7. d	16. b	
8. c	17. a	
9. d	18. b	

QTP

22. Proper shim coil adjustment improves B_o homogeneity, which in turn improves both spatial and contrast resolution.

23. The shim coils are located in the gantry next to the B_o coils. They are adjusted individually to make the B_o field more homogeneous.

Worksheet Number 12

1. d	10. d	19. a
2. d	11. b	20. d
3. c	12. d	21. d
4. d	13. b	
5. b	14. b	
6. d	15. c	
7. d	16. c	
8. c	17. c	
9. c	18. a	

QTP

22. The superimposed magnetic field gradient is approximately $1/1000$ (10^{-3}) of B_o.
23. This rhythmic thumping noise is produced by the mechanical vibration of the gradients coils as they slightly expand and contract during excitation.
24. RF bandwidth must be reduced.
25. Rise time is the time required for a gradient coil to reach its maximum current, therefore maximum magnetic field. It is measured in μs.
26. Oblique views result from energizing the three magnetic field gradient coils simultaneously.

Worksheet Number 13

1. c	10. d	19. b
2. d	11. b	
3. c	12. d	
4. a	13. b	
5. a	14. a	
6. c	15. c	
7. d	16. b	
8. d	17. b	
9. a	18. b	

QTP

20. MRI of osseous structures is selectively successful with bone containing enriched marrow. This is particularly useful in TMJ imaging.
21. The electrical leads of the surface coil may become frayed and heat excessive and may burn the patient. Coil wires, if overlapped during an MR examination, can short, causing superficial burns and an abortive scan.
22. Separate transmit and receive coils are used only for small field of view, high spatial resolution imaging. Surface coils are used to receive only.
23. Quadrature coils are used for head or body imaging. They detect the MR signal along orthogonal axes.
24. $\dfrac{120 \text{ mm}}{256 \text{ pixels}} = 0.5 \text{ mm/pixel}$

Worksheet Number 14

1. c	10. b	19. b
2. a	11. c	20. d
3. b	12. d	21. c
4. a	13. b	22. b
5. a	14. c	
6. d	15. a	
7. a	16. d	
8. c	17. a	
9. a	18. b	

23. A gauss meter or magnetometer is used to map the magnetic fringe field locally and in surrounding areas.
24. If service were remote, you would buy a permanent magnet imager.

Worksheet Number 15

1. d	10. c	19. d
2. d	11. b	20. a
3. d	12. c	21. d
4. a	13. d	22. b
5. c	14. c	23. 2, 1, 4, 3
6. b	15. a	
7. a	16. d	
8. c	17. d	
9. b	18. b	

QTP
24. MR rooms are shielded against RF with foil or meshed copper or aluminum to keep extraneous RF from other sources from entering the imaging room.
25. Permanent magnet imagers contain an enormous amount of iron to provide a return path for the magnetic field, which essentially contains the fringe field within the iron.

Worksheet Number 16

1. b	10. c
2. a	11. b
3. a	12. b
4. b	13. a
5. a	14. d
6. c	15. c
7. d	16. a
8. a	
9. b	

QTP
17. A modest change in temperature or humidity can create a host of electrical malfunctions, premature component failure, and increased system noise.
18. Helium, a gas found in natural deposits in Texas, Kansas, and New Mexico, must be separated by a specialized freezing process. Nitrogen is obtained by the fractional distillation of air, just like liquid oxygen.

Worksheet Number 17

1. c	10. b	19. b
2. c	11. a	20. b
3. d	12. b	21. a
4. a	13. c	22. d
5. c	14. c	23. b
6. d	15. d	24. a
7. a	16. c	25. b
8. c	17. d	26. b
9. c	18. b	27. c

QTP
28. Only elements containing odd A are capable of producing significant MR signals.
29. The gyromagnetic ratio of an element can be determined by measurement only. It cannot be calculated.
30. In 1 cc of tissue, which is approximately 1 g, there are an estimated 10^{23} hydrogen atoms. Therefore, approximately 10^{17} nuclei ($1/10^6 \times 10^{23} = 10^{17}$) contribute to the MR signal.
31. Coherence refers to the state of nuclear spins precessing in phase. They dephase with T2 relaxation time, and when completely dephased they are incoherent.

Worksheet Number 18

1. d
2. b
3. a
4. c
5. c
6. a
7. c
8. c
9. b
10. d
11. c
12. b
13. b
14. c
15. d
16. b

QTP

17. Forever!
18. One in a million spins will be aligned either with B_o or opposite B_o, with a slight excess of spins aligned with B_o. That is the low energy state.
19. The maximum intensity of an MRI signal occurs when spins are inphase or phase coherent.
20. Nuclear spins quickly dephase because of spin spin interaction. This is transverse (T2) relaxation.
21. Fat appears bright, especially on SDW and T1W images because of its high hydrogen content.

Worksheet Number 19

1. a
2. c
3. a
4. c
5. c
6. d
7. d
8. d
9. a
10. d
11. c
12. a
13. a
14. b
15. c
16. b
17. b
18. d
19. d

QTP

20. The homogeneity of the B_o field is varied by the applied magnetic field gradient, which in turn varies the Larmor frequency.
21. Magnetic field lines add vectorially, resulting in either a stronger, weaker, or directionally changed magnetic field.
22. Zero.
23. Spins are said to be saturated when $M_z = 0$ and $M_{xy} = M_o$. In this regard saturation is the opposite of equilibrium.
24. Fat, with its mobile proton and strong dipole-dipole interaction, produces the most intense MRI signal and brightest pixels. Cortical bone, cartilage, and fluid flow are at the other end of the scale.

Worksheet Number 20

1. c
2. d
3. b
4. d
5. a
6. a
7. b
8. c
9. c
10. b
11. c
12. b

QTP

13. M_o is parallel to B_o and therefore along the Z axis. It is perpendicular to the transverse, XY, plane.
14. The direction of the arrow represents the direction of net magnetization. The size of the arrow represents the magnitude of M.

1. c	10. c	19. a	28. b
2. c	11. d	20. a	29. c
3. c	12. d	21. a	
4. b	13. d	22. d	
5. a	14. a	23. b	
6. a	15. b	24. d	
7. d	16. b	25. b	
8. c	17. d	26. a	
9. a	18. b	27. c	

QTP

30. If imaging was done with a single frequency, the slice thickness would be too thin and the MR signal too low.
31. The bandwidth (BW) is the range of frequencies about the resonant frequency contained in the RF pulse.
32. The RF pulses are energized less than 1 ms, usually around 100μs.
33. Contiguous slices can be imaged sequentially; however, some RF will excite spins in an adjacent slice. That is crosstalk. It can be avoided by imaging with gaps between slices.
34. The rapid series of RF pulses at reduced flip angle will keep spins in a partially saturated state.

1. a	10. d	19. d
2. a	11. a	20. a
3. a	12. a	21. 4, 3, 2, 1
4. d	13. c	
5. a	14. d	
6. b	15. a	
7. a	16. d	
8. d	17. c	
9. b	18. a	

QTP

22. The simplest hydrogen isotope, ^{1}H, is the most important MR element in the body.
23. Both cortical bone and cartilage is imaged as dark, due to the lack of hydrogen and mobile protons.
24. Spin density (SD) is the number of protons available to produce the signal. This is analogous to the number of electrons (mAs) to produce x-rays. Double the SD or mAs and the respective signal production will double.
25. SD (spin density) is the number of protons in a given tissue voxel.
26. Contrast between tissues is directly proportional to SD in a SDW image. The SD of adjacent tissues also influences contrast directly in T1W and T2W images.

1. b	10. c	19. d
2. a	11. b	20. c
3. b	12. d	21. c
4. d	13. c	22. b
5. a	14. c	23. d
6. c	15. b	24. d
7. d	16. c	
8. c	17. d	
9. a	18. a	

QTP

25. The three intrinsic MRI parameters are spin density, longitudinal relaxation (T1), and transverse relaxation (T2).
26. Lattice refers to the molecular structure of the tissue in which the hydrogen resides.
27. Approximately five T1 relaxation times is required for return to equilibrium.
28. Relaxation times are measured in milliseconds (ms). One second = 1000 ms.
29. T1 = T2 only when referring to the relaxation time of pure water.

1.	c	10.	d	19.	c
2.	c	11.	a	20.	c
3.	d	12.	a	21.	d
4.	a	13.	c	22.	a
5.	c	14.	a	23.	b
6.	d	15.	a	24.	a
7.	d	16.	d		
8.	d	17.	a		
9.	c	18.	d		

QTP

25. SDW images produce a high contrast anatomical image. T2W images are usually low contrast, pathologically oriented.
26. T2* is the relaxation time of an FID. It is due principally to B_o inhomogeneities. T2* is always much shorter than T2.
27. The greater the tissue inhomogeneity the faster spin dephasing will occur because of bigger differences in spin spin interaction.
28. There is no effect. T2 is independent of B_o.

Worksheet Number 25

1.	a	10.	d	19.	c
2.	c	11.	a	20.	c
3.	b	12.	b		
4.	b	13.	d		
5.	a	14.	d		
6.	c	15.	b		
7.	c	16.	a		
8.	c	17.	c		
9.	d	18.	a		

QTP

21. T1 (with values of 100 s of ms) is always greater than T2 (with values of 10 s of ms).
22. That point in time where the transverse relaxation curves are farthest apart would exhibit the greatest contrast between adjacent tissues.
23. T2 relaxation occurs because of spin spin interactions within a molecule. T2* results from not only spin spin interactions but also because of B_o inhomogeneity and other regional influences.
24. T2 is related to the envelope of multiple spin echo amplitudes. T2* is related to the envelope of an FID.

Worksheet Number 26

1.	d	10.	a
2.	c	11.	b
3.	b	12.	c
4.	d	13.	c
5.	b	14.	a
6.	c	15.	c
7.	d	16.	d
8.	c		
9.	b		

QTP

17. T1 relaxation is always much slower than T2 relaxation.
18. The signal envelope is a theoretical line connecting the peaks of an MRI signal.
19. The math symbol $\geq$ means greater than or equal to.
20. T1 is lengthened with increasing B_o.
21. Increased signal amplitude always produces a bright image, but the TR/TE must be properly engaged to produce contrast.

1.	c	10.	d	19.	d
2.	b	11.	a	20.	c
3.	a	12.	b	21.	d
4.	d	13.	c	22.	a
5.	a	14.	c		
6.	c	15.	b		
7.	a	16.	c		
8.	a	17.	d		
9.	a	18.	b		

QTP

23. The simplest atom of hydrogen ^1H consists of a single proton in its nucleus and one orbiting k-electron. There are also more complex hydrogen atoms, deuterium ^2H and tritium ^3H. A water molecule (H_2O) consists of two hydrogen atoms bound to one oxygen atom.
24. Each nucleus has its own unique sensitivity value, the gyromagnetic ratio. It cannot be calculated as it is a GMIS value... God made it so!
25. The higher B_o, the more separated will be the spectral peaks in MRS. The peaks will each be more distin guishable.

1.	d	10.	a	19.	a
2.	c	11.	c	20.	a
3.	c	12.	b	21.	a
4.	d	13.	c	22.	d
5.	d	14.	c	23.	a
6.	c	15.	b	24.	b
7.	d	16.	c		
8.	b	17.	c		
9.	d	18.	c		

QTP

25. When two molecules such as fat/water experience a significant change in Larmor frequency, their dipole/ dipole interaction can cause an image misregistration, which is the chemical shift.
26. Chemical shift is measured in parts per million (ppm).
27. Tissue specificity is an image that demonstrates specific tissue structures one from another, such as lipids, edema, infection, normal vs abnormal tissue parenchyma, etc.
28. Unbound water produces a long relaxation time, due to its small molecular size and increased molecular motion. Fat consists of bound water and produces a short T1 relaxation time and moderate T2 relaxation time.
29. 3.5 ppm (4 T x 42 MHz/T) = 588 Hz.

1.	3, 1, 2, 4	10.	d	19.	d	28.	d	37.	d
2.	c	11.	d	20.	b	29.	c	38.	c
3.	b	12.	d	21.	d	30.	c	39.	d
4.	b	13.	b	22.	a	31.	d	40.	c
5.	d	14.	d	23.	c	32.	b	41.	c
6.	c	15.	c	24.	d	33.	b	42.	c
7.	d	16.	c	25.	c	34.	d	43.	b
8.	a	17.	c	26.	b	35.	a		
9.	b	18.	d	27.	d	36.	d		

QTP

44. To encode is to place a known signal or message onto an MR signal in order to decipher that signal.
45. The S/N is a ratio borrowed from electrical engineering, relating the intensity of an MRI signal to background noise. The greater the S/N the better the contrast resolution.
46. S/N is increased by increasing the number of signals acquired and averaging them. (Nex or Acq).

47. FOV is an abbreviation for the Field of View, or the clinical area being imaged. Conventionally, increased FOV refers to a large pixel size.
48. Image time does not change with a change in FOV.

Worksheet Number 30

1. d	10. c	19. c
2. b	11. a	20. b
3. 3, 4, 2, 1	12. d	21. b
4. b	13. c	22. c
5. a	14. d	23. c
6. d	15. c	
7. b	16. 2, 4, 3, 1	
8. a	17. a	
9. d	18. a	

QTP

24. As the magnetic field gradient is increased, the corresponding slice gets thinner and contrast resolution is reduced because there is less signal. In order to maintain constant S/N, scan time must be lengthened.
25. The MRI signals, SE and GE, are delayed for a time after the FID by either a 180^0 RF-refocussing pulse or a refocussing magnetic field gradient. Therefore the term echo is applied to reflect this delay in the signal production process.
26. An increase in FOV will decrease spatial resolution, due to the larger pixel size but may improve contrast resolution.
27. Large pixels/voxels result in better contrast because of increased SNR.

Worksheet Number 31

1. b	10. d	19. a
2. a	11. b	20. d
3. a	12. d	21. b
4. d	13. a	
5. d	14. d	
6. c	15. b	
7. b	16. c	
8. a	17. c	
9. c	18. c	

QTP

22. An artifact is an image detail or signal that does not represent a true feature of the object.
23. The frequency encoding axis is subject to chemical shift artifacts. This is typically the X or lateral axis.

Worksheet Number 32

1. d	10. b
2. d	11. b
3. d	12. c
4. d	13. d
5. a	14. c
6. a	
7. c	
8. b	
9. b	

QTP

15. An aliased image is caused by undersampling. The computer gets confused because the MRI signal has not been measured fast enough. The resultant image usually presents a wrap-around appearance.
16. The operator can reduce aliasing effects by being more selective in the choice of detector coils and/or FOV.
17. Truncation can be reduced by increasing the acquisition matrix size and selecting the proper reconstruction algorithm.

18. The matrix size is not changed with a change of FOV. However, the pixel size will be reduced with the magnification of smaller FOV and spatial resolution improved.
19. A magnified image resulting from reduced FOV has less contrast, but the spatial resolution is improved.

Worksheet Number 33

1. b	10. c	19. a
2. a	11. d	20. b
3. b	12. b	21. d
4. a	13. b	
5. b	14. d	
6. b	15. d	
7. c	16. b	
8. a	17. d	
9. c	18. b	

QTP
22. A possible correlation between MRI and X-ray parameters is as follows:

MRI	X-ray	Function
TE	kVp	principally controls contrast
TR	mAs	principally controls signal intensity

23. A short TR and short TE will produce a T1W image. A long TR and a long TE will produce a T2W image.
24. The T2W spin echo has less signal amplitude with more noise, but better contrast of pathology.
25. Short TR creates a partial saturation state because the net magnetization does not have time to return to equilibrium.
26. Scan time is directly proportional to the number of phase-encoding steps.

Worksheet Number 34

1. c	10. b	19. b
2. b	11. b	20. d
3. c	12. d	21. 1, 3, 4, 2
4. c	13. b	
5. b	14. b	
6. d	15. d	
7. d	16. b	
8. b	17. d	
9. a	18. d	

QTP
22. MRA has been very successful in imaging blood flow, thus lumen patency imaging. Hemorrhage is imaged because of the ferromagnetic iron normally found in blood.
23. The IR pulse sequence conventionally provides a heavily weighted T1 image and contrast reversal images where the spin density (SDW) becomes a dominant imaging factor.
24. The TR/TE times are changed to enhance image contrast.
25. Both TOF and PC images can be acquired in both 2D and 3D.
26. The influence of T2* is effectively removed by employing an 180^0 RF refocussing pulse.

212

Worksheet Number 35

1. b	10. a	19. d	28. d	37. a
2. a	11. b	20. b	29. c	38. a
3. b	12. a	21. a	30. b	39. d
4. a	13. a	22. d	31. a	40. c
5. d	14. d	23. a	32. b	41. b
6. b	15. b	24. a	33. b	42. a
7. b	16. d	25. c	34. a	43. a
8. c	17. b	26. d	35. b	
9. b	18. b	27. c	36. b	

QTP

44. An increase in data sampling reduces artifacts and improves spatial resolution and contrast resolution.
45. Yes, but by hand or with a calculator. It is a tedious exercise.

Worksheet Number 36

1. d	10. b	19. a	28. b	37. d
2. b	11. a	20. c	29. a	38. c
3. 2, 3, 4, 1	12. c	21. c	30. c	39. a
4. b	13. a	22. a	31. d	40. c
5. c	14. d	23. d	32. d	41. d
6. a	15. c	24. b	33. c	
7. a	16. c	25. c	34. b	
8. b	17. a	26. a	35. d	
9. c	18. c	27. a	36. d	

QTP

42. The phase and frequency of an MR signal is analyzed by the Fourier transformation process to determine spatial location.
43. If a second pulse sequence is initiated before spins have fully relaxed, there is a reduction in image signal and contrast because M_z is less than M_o.

Worksheet Number 37

1. 3, 4, 1, 2	10. b	19. b	28. c	37. b
2. c	11. c	20. d	29. b	
3. c	12. a	21. b	30. d	
4. c	13. c	22. d	31. d	
5. d	14. c	23. b	32. b	
6. c	15. a	24. c	33. b	
7. c	16. c	25. a	34. a	
8. c	17. a	26. c	35. d	
9. b	18. a	27. b	36. d	

QTP

38. Inversion recovery, with its $180^\circ/90^\circ/180^\circ$ RF pulse sequence, is used for T1-weighted images and may be used to reverse contrast.
39. There is no change in scan time.
40. Flow-related spins have not been subjected to the enormous refocussing RF pulse and therefore are more sensitive to minute changes.
41. FSE involves a series of rapidly applied 180° Rf pulses, each with a different phase-encoding gradient following the initial 90° RF pulse.
42. Longer TRs are a necessity for multiple spin echoes and multiple (volumetric) slice imaging.

1. b	10. d	19. a	
2. c	11. c	20. c	
3. b	12. b	21. a	
4. a	13. a	22. c	
5. c	14. d	23. c	
6. c	15. a		
7. a	16. c		
8. a	17. c		
9. d	18. d		

QTP

24. A series of 180° refocussing RF pulses, each with a different G_ϕ, is used in fast spin echo (FSE) imaging.
25. Inflow techniques rely on unsaturated spins flowing into the saturated slice, and this interaction with the departing flow spins in the slice creates distinct image contrast.
26. A presaturation pulse may be applied to either side of the slice. Some systems are equipped to presaturation entirely around a given ROI.
27. Whenever the diameter of the vessel decreases, the resistance will correspondingly increase, thus reducing blood flow velocity. The often unsuspected presence of stenosis, atherosclerosis, or aneurysm will alter blood flow velocity.
28. Fast scanning is generally SDW and T2W, becoming more T1W with larger flip angles.

Worksheet Number 39

1. d	10. c	19. b
2. b	11. d	20. c
3. b	12. c	
4. c.	13. a	
5. c	14. c	
6. d	15. c	
7. c	16. d	
8. d	17. c	
9. c	18. d	

QTP

21. Most of the body's water is in solution and therefore unbound. When water is bound to larger macromolecules, such as proteins, relaxation time is reduced, producing higher signal on most sequence.
22. Bipolar means two poles and refers to the DC current applied first in one direction and then in the opposite direction. This creates a changing, bipolar magnetic field.
23. Long TR enables the stationary tissues to become unsaturated. The excited blood may flow out of the slice before it can be refocussed by the gradient.
24. The two basic MRA pulse sequences are time of flight (TOF) and phase contrast (PC).
25. As the flip angle is reduced, the S/N is reduced.

Worksheet Number 40

1. a	10. d	19. b	28. d
2. d	11. a	20. b	29. a
3. b	12. d	21. b	30. a
4. c	13. d	22. c	31. c
5. a	14. c	23. c	32. d
6. d	15. a	24. d	33. a
7. c	16. d	25. b	34. c
8. b	17. c	26. c	
9. b	18. d	27. b	

QTP

35. There are 25.4 mm/inch and therefore $25.4 \div 3.5 = 7.3$ or 7 complete slices.
36. The two principle parameters governing spatial resolution are the number of phase-encoding signal acquisitions and the field of view (FOV).

37. In 3D imaging the entire volume is RF excited rather than sequential slice excitation as in 2D imaging.
38. There are various trade-off factors involving a change in the pixel/voxel size, such as:

$$\text{Pixel/voxel} \downarrow = \uparrow \text{spatial resolution}$$
$$= \downarrow \text{contrast resolution}$$
$$= \downarrow \text{S/N}$$

39. Magnetic field gradients function under the same principle and therefore are often interchanged—primarily to remove/reduce artifacts or to change to a different imaging plane.

Worksheet Number 41

1. d	10. d	19. d	28. c
2. a	11. d	20. d	29. a
3. c	12. b	21. d	30. a
4. a	13. a	22. b	31. a
5. c	14. d	23. c	32. b
6. c	15. b	24. b	
7. b	16. b	25. c	
8. b	17. a	26. d	
9. a	18. c	27. c	

QTP

33. The signal amplitude at the mid-point of the spin echo is highest because spins are in phase.
34. G_R is energized during the time of any MR signal and remains on while a signal is being acquired or read.
35. A multispin echo pulse sequence produces images with a distinctly different contrast rendition and no increase in scan time.
36. The TOF method tags unsaturated bolus at one position and identifies it as another where it replaces the original saturated blood.
37. Phase contrast (PC) imaging quantitatively measures and records the characteristics of laminar blood flow by the changes in its phase of spins as they move through a gradient.

Worksheet Number 42

1. c	10. a	19. a
2. d	11. b	20. d
3. 1, 4, 2, 3	12. d	21. b
4. c	13. d	22. b
5. c	14. 2, 4, 1, 3	
6. c	15. a	
7. b	16. a	
8. c	17. c	
9. c	18. 2, 3, 4, 1	

QTP

23. Transverse - top to bottom
    Coronal - front to back
    Sagittal - side to side
24. Bone marrow is rich with mobile protons (high spin density) and appears bright on most images.
25. The human eye can distinguish approximately 20 different shades of gray.
26. A magnified image reflects smaller pixel size, reduced contrast, and improved spatial resolution.

Worksheet Number 43

1. a	10. c
2. a	11. d
3. c	12. c
4. b	
5. a	
6. d	
7. b	
8. a	
9. a	

13. Unlike CT, MRI cannot image bone because there is very little mobile hydrogen. Consequently there are no artifacts.
14. Cartilage is dark on MRI. When contrasted to hydrogen enriched bone marrow, cartilage appears very hypointense.
15. The more shades of gray, the better. Proper postprocessing, windowing, and leveling should allow visualization of all shades of gray.
16. Scan Time = TR x NEX x NP = 3000 x 2 x 256 = 1,536,000 ms = 1,536 s = 25.6 min.
17. A change in the T1 relaxation time has no effect on imaging time. TR, NEX, and the number of phase-encoding steps determine imaging time.

Worksheet Number 44

1. a	13. b	25. b	37. c	49. a
2. d	14. c	26. d	38. c	50. a
3. a	15. b	27. c	39. a	51. a
4. c	16. d	28. b	40. a	52. a
5. b	17. a	29. c	41. d	53. d
6. c	18. b	30. 4, 3, 2, 1	42. b	54. d
7. d	19. c	31. c	43. a	55. d
8. d	20. d	32. d	44. d	56. b
9. a	21. a	33. d	45. a	57. a
10. a	22. c	34. d	46. c	58. d
11. c	23. b	35. d	47. b	
12. c	24. c	36. a	48. b	

59. Hypointense describes a gray-dark tissue.
60. Spin density–weighted images are referred to as anatomical because they are relatively high contrast.
61. Signal intensity reflects the amount of transverse magnetization (M_{xy}) in tissue at the time of sampling. Image contrast reflects the relative difference in signal intensity between adjacent tissues.
62. A low S/N image appears grainy with low contrast.

Worksheet Number 45

1. b	10. 1	19. 20	28. 8
2. 9	11. 10	20. 16	29. 5
3. 4	12. 13	21. 6	30. 2
4. 12	13. 8	22. 3	31. 3
5. 21	14. 5	23. 22	32. 1
6. 18	15. 23	24. 14	33. 6
7. 2	16. 19	25. b	
8. 7	17. 15	26. 7	
9. 17	18. 11	27. 4	

Worksheet Number 46

1. c	13. b	23. 7	33. 4
2. 5	14. 12	24. 4	34. 5
3. 8	15. 10	25. 13	
4. 9	16. 11	26. 2	
5. 10	17. 1	27. c	
6. 2	18. 5	28. 6	
7. 3	19. 8	29. 2	
8. 7	20. 9	30. 7	
9. 6	21. 6	31. 1	
10. 4	22. 3	32. 3	
11. 1			

12. cochlear nerve, facial nerve, and the two divisions of the vestibular nerve

Worksheet Number 47

1. 6
2. 4
3. 1
4. 3
5. 5
6. 2
7. d
8. 6
9. 9
10. 7
11. 11
12. 2
13. 4
14. 3
15. 5
16. 8
17. 10
18. 1
19. anterior inferior
    third ventricle
20. b
21. d

Worksheet Number 48

1. d
2. 2
3. 1
4. 3
5. time-of-flight
6. 3
7. 1
8. 4
9. 2
10. left subclavian artery
11. 2
12. 4
13. 1
14. 3
15. brachiocephalic artery

Worksheet Number 49

1. b
2. 2
3. 3
4. 4
5. 5
6. 1
7. a
8. 2
9. 3
10. 1
11. 4
12. 1
13. 4
14. 3
15. 2

Worksheet Number 50

1. 1
2. 9
3. 6
4. 7
5. 8
6. 5
7. 4
8. C3-4 interspace
9. C7
10. c
11. C2
12. C3-4 interspace
13. C5
14. cerebrospinal fluid
15. spinal cord
16. spinous process
17. 6
18. 5
19. 1
20. 4
21. 3
22. 2
23. neural foramen

Worksheet Number 51

1. b
2. 2
3. 5
4. 1
5. 4
6. 3
7. c
8. 2
9. 5
10. 6
11. 1
12. 7
13. 4
14. 3
15. transverse foramen
16. atlantoaxial joint
17. 5
18. 7
19. 4
20. 1
21. 3
22. 6
23. vertebral bodies, pedicles, and facets

Worksheet Number 52

1. b
2. 5
3. 2
4. 3
5. 6
6. 4
7. 1
8. c
9. high water content

10. 2
11. 4
12. 5
13. 3
14. 1
15. 6
16. 7
17. 2
18. 3

19. 4
20. 5
21. 1
22. b
23. 5
24. 6
25. 2
26. 8
27. 1

28. 4
29. 3
30. 7

Worksheet Number 53

1. b
2. 1
3. 6
4. 7
5. 5
6. L3-4 interspace
7. L2
8. S1
9. c

10. L3
11. L4-5 interspace
12. S1
13. 7
14. 5
15. 4
16. 6
17. 4
18. 6

19. 1
20. 5
21. 3
22. 2

Worksheet Number 54

1. b
2. 5
3. 4
4. 1
5. 2
6. 3
7. 3
8. 8
9. 5

10. 6
11. 1
12. 2
13. 4
14. 7
15. c
16. 5
17. 7
18. 2

19. 4
20. 3
21. 6
22. 1
23. c
24. 6
25. 5
26. 3
27. 2

28. 4
29. 1
30. 7

Worksheet Number 55

1. 5
2. 6
3. 3
4. 7
5. 4
6. 1
7. 2
8. 7
9. 8

10. 6
11. 4
12. 3
13. 1
14. 2
15. 5
16. the first image
17. b
18. c

Worksheet Number 56

1.	4	10.	5
2.	7	11.	3
3.	8	12.	8
4.	5	13.	6
5.	6	14.	4
6.	1	15.	7
7.	3	16.	2
8.	2	17.	diastole
9.	1	18.	the second image

Worksheet Number 57

1.	3	10.	1
2.	6	11.	3
3.	8	12.	2
4.	5	13.	6
5.	2	14.	5
6.	7	15.	4
7.	9		
8.	4		
9.	1		

Worksheet Number 58

1.	3	13.	5	24.	c
2.	1	14.	6		
3.	4	15.	3		
4.	2	16.	1		
5.	5	17.	4		
6.	4	18.	2		
7.	2	19.	2		
8.	5	20.	3		
9.	3	21.	1		
10.	1	22.	4		
11.	b	23.	a		

12. To destroy the signal from fluid that may be isointense with contrast-enhanced tissues.

Worksheet Number 59

1.	9	10.	6	19.	2	28.	9
2.	8	11.	7	20.	c	29.	7
3.	3	12.	6	21.	1	30.	5
4.	1	13.	1	22.	2	31.	8
5.	7	14.	5	23.	6	32.	b
6.	10	15.	4	24.	4	33.	a
7.	5	16.	3	25.	10	34.	a
8.	4	17.	8	26.	11		
9.	2	18.	9	27.	3		

Worksheet Number 60

1.	c	10.	4	19.	3	28.	3
2.	5	11.	7	20.	6	29.	b
3.	2	12.	b	21.	2		
4.	8	13.	8	22.	9		
5.	1	14.	5	23.	a		
6.	6	15.	4	24.	1		
7.	9	16.	10	25.	2		
8.	3	17.	7	26.	5		
9.	10	18.	1	27.	4		

Worksheet Number 61

1.	b	10.	1
2.	2	11.	2
3.	1	12.	3
4.	4	13.	5
5.	6	14.	4
6.	3		
7.	7		
8.	5		
9.	b		

Worksheet Number 62

1.	a	10.	4	19.	c
2.	c	11.	5	20.	c
3.	c	12.	1		
4.	d	13.	b		
5.	TMJ capsule	14.	5		
6.	mandibular condyle	15.	2		
		16.	3		
7.	c	17.	1		
8.	2	18.	4		
9.	3				

Worksheet Number 63

1.	b	10.	1	19.	4
2.	2	11.	3	20.	4
3.	5	12.	2	21.	3
4.	6	13.	deltoid muscle	22.	2
5.	4	14.	a	23.	5
6.	7	15.	a	24.	1
7.	1	16.	3	25.	supraspinatous, infraspinatous, subscapularis, teres minor
8.	3	17.	2		
9.	c	18.	1		

Worksheet Number 64

1.	b	10.	3	19.	7
2.	3	11.	1	20.	a
3.	1	12.	c		
4.	4	13.	1		
5.	5	14.	6		
6.	2	15.	3		
7.	a	16.	4		
8.	4	17.	5		
9.	2	18.	2		

Worksheet Number 65

1. b	10. 3	19. 2	28. c
2. 2	11. 6	20. 1	29. 2
3. 1	12. 8	21. 4	30. 3
4. 7	13. b	22. 3	31. 1
5. 5	14. 4	23. 3	32. 4
6. 11	15. 1	24. 4	33. a
7. 9	16. 3	25. 5	34. b
8. 10	17. flexor digitorum	26. 1	
9. 4	18. a	27. 2	

Worksheet Number 66

1. b	10. 5	19. 6	28. 1
2. b	11. 4	20. 3	
3. 3	12. 1	21. 7	
4. 7	13. a	22. 4	
5. 10	14. 2	23. c	
6. 9	15. 5	24. 2	
7. 6	16. 1	25. 3	
8. 8	17. 8	26. 5	
9. 2	18. 9	27. 4	

Worksheet Number 67

1. 5	10. 3	19. 6
2. 4	11. 4	20. 8
3. 3	12. 2	21. 4
4. 2	13. 5	22. 2
5. 6	14. 4	23. 3
6. 1	15. 1	24. 1
7. 7	16. 2	25. 9
8. 1	17. 3	26. 7
9. 5	18. 5	

Worksheet Number 68

1. c	10. 5	19. navicular	28. 7
2. 6	11. b	20. talus	29. 9
3. 8	12. 6	21. calcaneous	30. 5
4. 9	13. 4	22. Achilles tendon	31. 8
5. 4	14. 1	23. a	32. 4
6. 3	15. 5	24. 3	
7. 7	16. 2	25. 2	
8. 2	17. 3	26. 6	
9. 1	18. a	27. 1	

Worksheet Number 69

1. c	10. c	19. a	28. c	37. b
2. b	11. d	20. d	29. b	38. c
3. c	12. a	21. a	30. a	39. a
4. a	13. d	22. b	31. c	40. d
5. d	14. b	23. a	32. b	
6. a	15. c	24. c	33. c	
7. b	16. d	25. b	34. d	
8. c	17. b	26. a	35. c	
9. a	18. c	27. a	36. c	

QTP

41. DTPA (diethylenetriaminepenteta acetic acid) is a "detoxifier" that neutralizes the metallic properties of the paramagnetic gadolinium.
42. Gadolinium has seven unpaired electrons and nine binding sites, thus it is very paramagnetic.
43. Gd-DTPA is most effective in enhancing contrast of tumors, infection, infarction, and inflammation.
44. Just as protons do, electrons spin on an imaginary axis either clockwise or counterclockwise. An odd number of electrons in a given shell will result in one without an opposite spinning partner.

Worksheet Number 70

1. a	10. d	19. a	28. a
2. d	11. c	20. b	29. d
3. c	12. b	21. b	30. 4, 1, 2, 3
4. a	13. c	22. d	31. c
5. b	14. d	23. b	32. d
6. b	15. a	24. c	
7. d	16. d	25. c	
8. d	17. b	26. b	
9. a	18. d	27. a	

QTP

33. Yes. Though a permanent magnet imager has a vertical magnetic field when a ferromagnetic object is brought very close to the imager, it can exert a very strong projectile influence.
34. SAR is measured in W/kg.
35. The most important factor that could cause an imaging procedure to exceed the FDA SAR guidelines is the number and duration of RF pulses.

Worksheet Number 71

1. d	10. a
2. b	11. b
3. b	12. b
4. b	13. b
5. b	14. b
6. d	
7. c	
8. a	
9. c	

QTP

15. Stainless steel is non-ferromagnetic; however, it often contains a ferromagnetic alloy.
16. The RF energy absorbed can elevate body temperature.

Worksheet Number 72

1. b	10. d
2. b	11. a
3. d	12. c
4. c	13. a
5. c	
6. a	
7. b	
8. b	
9. c	

QTP

14. $K = {}^{\circ}C + 273$

$$K = \frac{{}^{\circ}F - 32}{1.8} + 273$$

15. Gold is not ferromagnetic, but the stem of pins, necklaces, and earrings may be. There have been reported cases where earrings have been magnetically pulled off the operator's ear; the gold portion falls harmlessly to the floor, and the ferromagnetic stem lodges in the gantry.
16. Special glasses are available for the patient to wear during the examination that creates the illusion to the patient that the gantry bore is larger and therefore less confining. Also, music, TV, and special fragrances are being effectively used to reduce patient anxiety.
17. Vaporization of the cryogens as during a quench can reduce the oxygen level in room air.

Worksheet Number 73

1.	a	10.	d	19.	d
2.	a	11.	a	20.	b
3.	c	12.	c	21.	c
4.	d	13.	d		
5.	d	14.	c		
6.	d	15.	b		
7.	c	16.	b		
8.	d	17.	a		
9.	c	18.	d		

QTP

22. Surgical clips can create regional ghosting artifacts or absence of signal.
23. The MR operator should routinely check surface coils for electrical integrity. Never loop coil leads.
24. SAR is an acronym for "specific absorption rate." It is measured in W/kg andrelated to RF energy disposition in tissue.
25. Prosthetic implants are usually visualized as noise or a signal void.

Worksheet Number 74

1.	c	10.	d	19.	b	28.	d
2.	a	11.	b	20.	a	29.	d
3.	b	12.	a	21.	b	30.	b
4.	d	13.	b	22.	a		
5.	b	14.	a	23.	c		
6.	a	15.	d	24.	c		
7.	d	16.	a	25.	d		
8.	d	17.	b	26.	b		
9.	c	18.	c	27.	a		

QTP

31. Generally, when scan time is reduced for whatever reason, there is a trade-off with reduced signal-to-noise ratio and therefore a reduction in image quality.
32. There are elaborate references available to determine whether a particular brand of clip or prosthesis is ferromagnetic.
33. Dental fillings will generally create regional ghosting patterns or absence of signal when imaging the head, including the occlusal area.
34. CT images are basically high contrast bone/trauma oriented, whereas MRI is primarily related to tissue contrast. At the present time CT is less vulnerable to motion artifacts.
35. The operator will first take a scout image to assure that the presentation slice is oriented to the vessel of interest. The scout image reveals the presaturation slice.

1. d	10. c
2. d	11. c
3. b	12. c
4. d	13. b
5. d	14. d
6. b	15. b
7. c	
8. d	
9. d	

QTP

16. Apparently females experience less claustrophobia than males.

17. A radiographic examination may be necessary to rule out the presence of metallic slivers in the face or eyes. Such incidents have been reported to cause hemorrhaging, loss of sight, and even death.

18. USFDA is an abbreviation for the U.S. Food and Drug Administration. The U.S. Center for Devices and Radiation Health is a part of the USFDA. This is the federal agency that registers the safety of MRI devices.

Appendix B

Practice Exam A

☐ **PATIENT CARE AND MRI SAFETY**

1. Paramagnetic contrast agents are most effective with _____ -weighted pulse sequences.

   a. T1
   b. T2
   c. spin density
   d. electron density

2. MRI contrast agents principally work through a reduction in:

   a. spin density
   b. electron density
   c. relaxation times
   d. flow phenomena

3. Use of the chelating agent DTPA is effective because it:
   (1) increases spin density
   (2) lowers toxicity
   (3) changes relaxation time
   (4) increases elimination

   a. 1, 2, and 3
   b. 1 and 3
   c. 2 and 4
   d. 4

4. The main potential for a biologic response from RF is:

   a. tissue heating
   b. polarization
   c. induction of currents
   d. suppression of relaxation time

5. The interaction between transient magnetic fields and tissue is due to:

   a. radiation absorption
   b. electromagnetic induction
   c. electromagnetic radiation
   d. radiation induction

6. Some biologic responses have been reported in subjects imaged with 4 T research imagers. These include:
   (1) metallic taste
   (2) twitching
   (3) disequilibrium
   (4) magnetophosphene induction

   a. 1, 2, and 3
   b. 1 and 3
   c. 2 and 4
   d. all are correct

7. Pacemakers can be interrupted at static magnetic fields of approximately:

   a. 2 mT
   b. 5 mT
   c. 10 mT
   d. 50 mT

8. A patient with a history of intraorbital metal can be imaged if:

   a. the metal is identified radiographically
   b. the metal is identified fluoroscopically
   c. the metal is considered nonmagnetic
   d. never

225

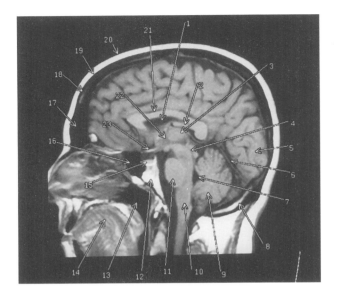

9. What type of contrast is dominant in this sagittal image?

   a. spin density   c. T2
   b. T1   d. T2*

10. Which arrow points to the fornix? _____

11. Which arrow points to the medulla oblongata? _____

Questions 12 and 13 refer to the figure below.

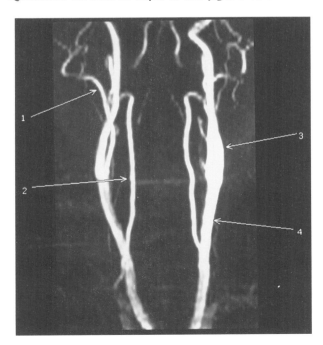

12. Which arrow points to the external carotid artery? _____

13. Which arrow points to the common carotid artery? _____

Questions 14 to 16 refer to the following figure.

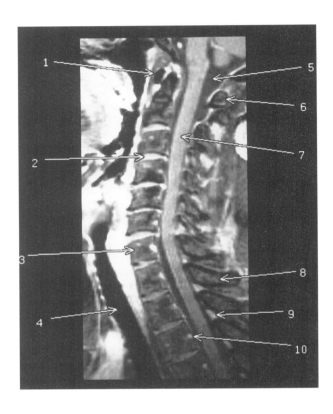

14. Which arrow points to the anterior arch of C1? _____

15. Which arrow points to the spinal cord? _____

16. Which arrow points to the trachea? _____

Questions 17 to 19 refer to the following figure.

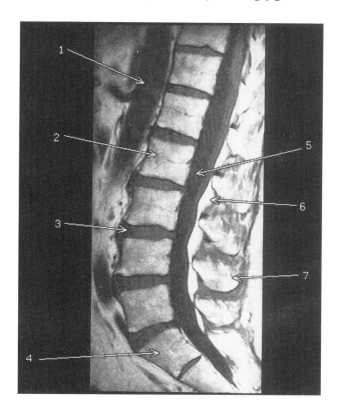

17. Which arrow points to the aorta? _____

18. Which arrow points to the spinous process? _____

19. Which arrow points to the subarachnoid space? _____

Questions 20 to 22 refer to the following figure.

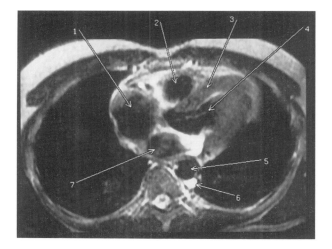

20. Which arrow points to the hemiazygos vein? _____

21. Which arrow points to the left atrium? _____

22. Which arrow points to the right ventricle? _____

Questions 23 and 24 refer to the figure below.

23. Which arrow points to the breast parenchyma? _____

24. Which arrow points to the silicone implant? _____

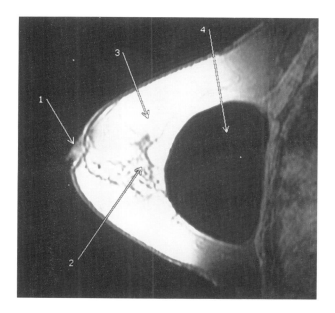

Questions 25 to 27 refer to the following figure.

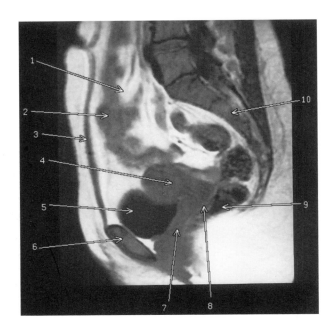

25. The structures demonstrated in this image are in what anatomical plane?

    a. transverse
    b. sagittal
    c. coronal
    d. oblique

26. Which arrow points to the cervix? _____

27. Which arrow points to the rectus abdominus muscle? _____

Questions 28 to 30 refer to the figure below.

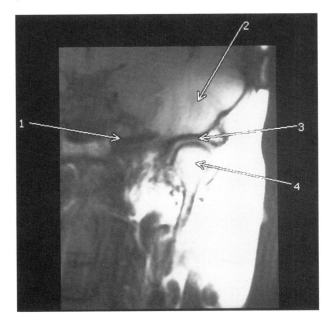

28. The structures demonstrated in this image are in what anatomical plane?

    a. transverse
    b. sagittal
    c. coronal
    d. oblique

29. Arrow #1 points to the:

    a. auditory nerve
    b. internal auditory canal
    c. internal carotid artery
    d. middle cerebral artery

30. Arrow #2 points to the:

    a. frontal lobe
    b. occipital lobe
    c. parietal lobe
    d. temporal lobe

Questions 31 and 32 refer to the following figure.

31. The structures demonstrated in this image are in what anatomical plane?

    a. transverse
    b. sagittal
    c. coronal
    d. oblique

32. Which arrow points to the olecranon? _____

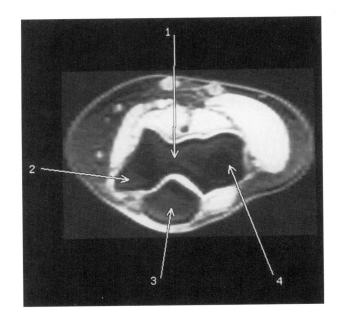

Questions 33 and 34 refer to the following figure.

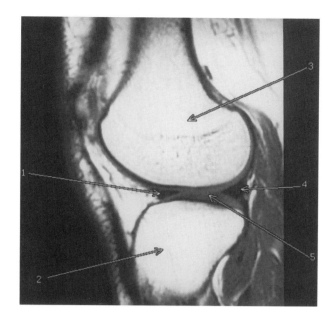

33. Which arrow points to the articular cartilage? _____

34. Which arrow points to the posterior lateral meniscus? _____

☐ DATA ACQUISITION AND PROCESSING

35. Following a 180° RF pulse, the signal received from the patient is:

    a. flat
    c. a spin echo
    b. a free induction decay
    d. a gradient echo

36. Which of the following pulse sequences will produce a spin echo?

    a. 90°...90°...90°...
    c. 180°...180°...180°...
    b. 90°...180°...90°...180°...
    d. 180°...90°...180°...90°...

37. As M_{xy} relaxes to zero:
    (1) signal intensity decreases
    (2) signal intensity increases
    (3) an FID is produced
    (4) nothing happens

    a. 1, 2, and 3   c. 2 and 4
    b. 1 and 3   d. all are correct

38. Control of TE is exercised by control of:

    a. the 90° RF pulse   c. the T1 relaxation time
    b. the 180° RF pulse   d. the T2 relaxation time

39. Which of the diagrams in the following figure symbolizes a varying phase-encoding gradient pulse?

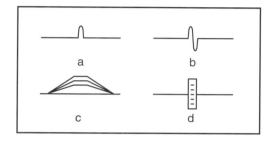

40. The Fourier transformation of a spin echo results in information in the:

    a. time domain   c. length domain
    b. frequency domain   d. volume domain

41. In MRI smooth objects are represented by:

    a. zero frequency
    c. high frequencies
    b. low frequencies
    d. a wide range of frequencies

42. When a spin echo is Fourier transformed (see the figure below), the result will appear as:

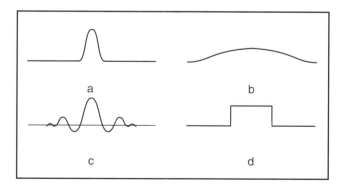

43. If the sampling rate of an MR signal is insufficient, the result is an artifact called:

   a. truncation
   b. Gibbs phenomena
   c. magnetic susceptibility
   d. aliasing

44. The mathematical tool used to analyze the frequency content of an object is the:

   a. induction transform
   c. imaginary number rule
   b. Fourier transform
   d. Cartesian number rule

45. The trajectory in k-space refers to:

   a. each X and Y point
   b. each angle and distance
   c. the method of sampling the spatial frequency domain
   d. the method of sampling the temporal frequency domain

46. Most images have more signal at:
   (1) high spin density
   (2) low spin density
   (3) low spatial frequencies
   (4) high spatial frequencies

   a. 1, 2, and 3
   b. 1 and 3
   c. 2 and 4
   d. 4

47. In FSE the zero order spin echo follows the:

   a. first 180⁰ RF pulse
   b. last 180⁰ RF pulse
   c. weakest phase-encoding gradient pulse
   d. strongest phase-encoding gradient pulse

48. Partial Fourier imaging is possible because of:

   a. long repetition times
   b. long echo times
   c. high magnetic field strengths
   d. Hermitian symmetry

49. T2* is shorter than T2 principally because of:

   a. differences in T1
   b. differences in TI
   c. the influence of reversible magnetic field inhomogeneities
   d. the influence of irreversible magnetic field inhomogeneities

50. For completeness an MR pulse sequence diagram should contain at least _____ lines of information.

   a. one
   b. three
   c. five
   d. seven

51. Which of the drawings in the following figure corresponds to the coordinate system used for vector diagrams?

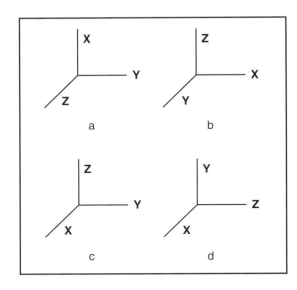

52. While the phase-encoding gradient is pulsed with different amplitude for each signal acquisition, the frequency-encoding gradient is:
   (1) pulsed with different amplitude also
   (2) pulsed with the same amplitude
   (3) on during the RF pulse
   (4) on during signal acquisition

   a. 1, 2, and 3
   b. 1 and 3
   c. 2 and 4
   d. 4

53. Magnetic field gradients are made more intense by:

   a. leaving them on longer
   b. pulsing the gradient coil
   c. applying a higher voltage to the gradient coil
   d. running more current through the gradient coil

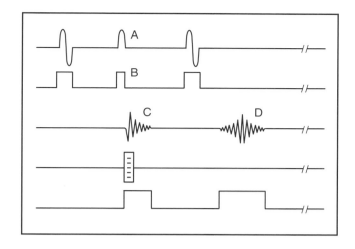

54. Which letter in the pulse sequence in the above figure represents a 90° RF pulse?

    a. A   c. C
    b. B   d. D

55. Which of the following influence the character of an MRI pixel?
  (1) electron density
  (2) spin density
  (3) optical density
  (4) motion

    a. 1, 2, and 3   c. 2 and 4
    b. 1 and 3   d. all are correct

56. Which letter in the following figure represents a voxel?

    a. A   c. C
    b. B   d. D

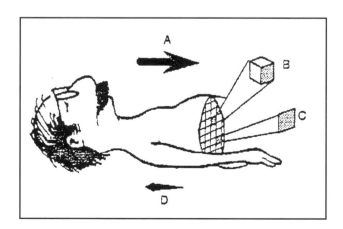

57. Which has the shortest relaxation time (see the figure below)?

    a. A   c. C
    b. B   d. D

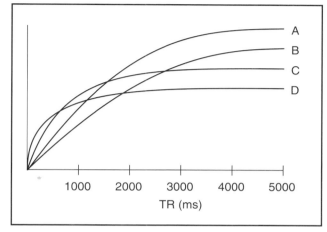

58. The principle secondary MRI parameters that affect pixel character are:
  (1) chemical shift
  (2) paramagnetic materials
  (3) magnetic susceptibility
  (4) motion

    a. 1, 2, and 3   c. 2 and 4
    b. 1 and 3   d. all are correct

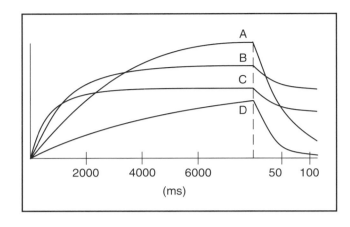

59. Which tissue in the above figure has the shortest T1 relaxation time?

a. A   c. C
b. B   d. D

60. Which letter in the figure below represents the spin echo pulse sequence combination of TR and TE that will result in a spin density–weighted image?

a. A   c. C
b. B   d. D

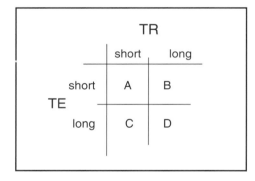

61. When MR images are rendered in color, the primary colors employed are:

a. blue, green, and yellow
b. green, yellow, and red
c. red, blue, and yellow
d. blue, green, and red

62. Which of the four tissues in the figure below has the shortest spin spin relaxation time?

a. A   c. C
b. B   d. D

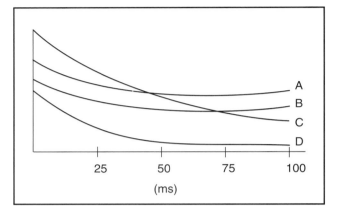

63. A partial saturation image made with a short repetition time is most likely a:

a. spin density–weighted image
b. T1 weighted image
c. T2 weighted image
d. a pure image

64. When post-processing an MR image, ROI stands for:
(1) region of interest
(2) relaxation on inversion
(3) a method of obtaining quantitative data
(4) a method of observing qualitative change

a. 1, 2, and 3   c. 2 and 4
b. 1 and 3   d. 4

65. Cones of the human retina are:

a. concentrated at the center of the retina
b. most numerous on the periphery of the retina
c. all at the fovea centralis
d. uniformly distributed on the retina

❒ PHYSICAL PRINCIPLES OF IMAGE FORMATION

66. Which of the following image modalities has best contrast resolution?

a. radioisotope image
b. radiography
c. computed tomography
d. magnetic resonance imaging

67. A spinning gyroscope:

    a. becomes polarized
    b. shows net magnetization
    c. induces a magnetic field
    d. has angular momentum

68. Induction refers to:

    a. a magnetic field generated by rotation
    b. precession in a magnetic field
    c. transfer of energy without touching
    d. interaction of electromagnetic radiation

69. Power is defined as:

    a. energy per unit mass
    b. energy per unit charge
    c. the rate of energy use
    d. the rate of coulomb flow

70. The most intense magnetic field of an electromagnet is:

    a. around the current carrying wire
    b. just off the ends
    c. lateral to the coil
    d. on the axis of the coil

71. An MR imaging room must be shielded to:

    a. keep electromagnetic radiation in the room
    b. keep electromagnetic radiation out of the room
    c. reduce acoustic interference
    d. reduce ionizing radiation levels

72. A feature of MRI electromagnets not found in permanent magnet systems is/are the:
    (1) gantry
    (2) gradient coils
    (3) shim coils
    (4) cooling system

    a. 1, 2, and 3   c. 2 and 4
    b. 1 and 3   d. 4

73. The purpose of a pole face is to:

    a. intensify the B_o field
    b. intensify the magnetic field gradients
    c. improve B_o homogeneity
    d. improve magnetic field gradient homogeneity

74. A 1.5 T magnet has a field homogeneity of ± 3 μT. This is equivalent to

    a. ± 2 ppm   c. ± 20 ppm
    b. ± 3 ppm   d. ± 30 ppm

75. Which of the drawings in the following figure represents the simplest MRI RF probe?

    a. A   c. C
    b. B   d. D

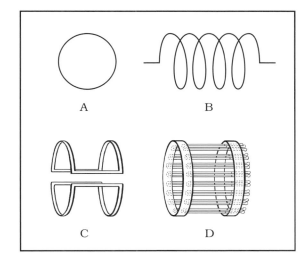

76. With reference to the magnets illustrated in the figure below, which uses the most electricity?

    a. A   c. C
    b. B   d. D

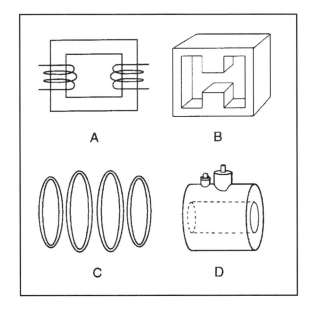

77. The room for storing cryogens must be:

    a. refrigerated   c. RF protected
    b. secured   d. magnetic field protected

78. Quantum mechanics is that branch of physics that describes very:

    a. large objects   c. high energies
    b. small objects   d. low energies

79. M_o is inversely proportional to:

    a. spin density
    b. gyromagnetic ratio
    c. B
    d. T

80. Which of the following vector diagrams in represents a 90^0 RF pulse?

    a. A   c. C
    b. B   d. D

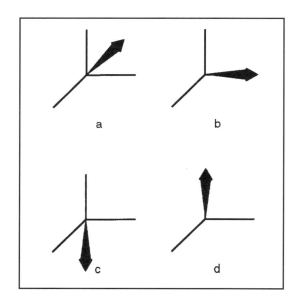

81. Spin density is most closely associated with a point at (refer to the figure below):

    a. A   c. C
    b. B   d. D

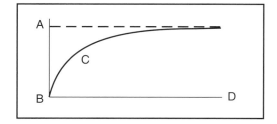

82. Spin spin relaxation represents relaxation:
    (1) in the M_{xy} plane
    (2) along the M_o axis
    (3) transverse to the M_o axis
    (4) transverse to the M_{xy} plane

    a. 1, 2, and 3   c. 2 and 4
    b. 1 and 3   d. 4

83. Magnetization of tissue along the Z axis cannot be measured directly because:
    (1) the B_o field is too intense
    (2) M_{xy} is too small
    (3) M_z is too small
    (4) T1 relaxation time is too short

    a. 1, 2, and 3   c. 2 and 4
    b. 1 and 3   d. 4

84. The carbon nucleus investigated for in vivo NMR spectroscopy is:

    a. C-10   c. C-12
    b. C-11   d. C-13

85. A good example of sampling a continous signal is:

    a. the detection of an MRI signal
    b. the detection of a video signal
    c. the display of an MRI image
    d. the display of a video image

86. The dynamic range of an MR image is described as 8 bits deep. How many bytes is required for each pixel?

    a. 1   c. 4
    b. 2   d. 8

87. Images that are particularly sensitive to magnetic field inhomogeneities are:
    (1) those produced by surface coils
    (2) those produced by the body coil
    (3) GE images
    (4) SE images

    a. 1, 2, and 3   c. 2 and 4
    b. 1 and 3   d. all are correct

Appendix C

Practice Exam B

☐ **PATIENT CARE AND MRI SAFETY**

1. Relaxation centers are regions of:

    a. increased spin density
    b. increased magnetization
    c. reduced T1 relaxation
    d. reduced T2 relaxation

2. Paramagnetism is due to:

    a. high atomic number
    b. varying electron density
    c. unpaired orbital electrons
    d. odd numbers of nucleons

3. Paramagnetic contrast agents enhance brain tumors by:

    a. changing spin density
    b. crossing the blood-brain barrier
    c. increasing T1 relaxation time
    d. increasing T2 relaxation time

4. The suspected biologic effect of the RF field occurs principally because of:

    a. induced currents   c. polarization
    b. tissue heating   d. relaxation

5. The suspected biologic effect of the static magnetic field occurs principally because of:

    a. induced currents   c. polarization
    b. tissue heating   d. relaxation

6. Human responses have been observed following exposure to:
    (1) transient magnetic fields
    (2) static magnetic fields
    (3) RF emissions
    (4) none of the above

    a. 1, 2, and 3   c. 2 and 4
    b. 1 and 3   d. 4

7. Earplugs should be used for hearing protection since gradient switching can produce sound levels up to approximately:

    a. 25 dB   c. 100 dB
    b. 50 dB   d. 150 dB

8. The pregnant patient:

    a. should not be imaged with MRI
    b. should not be imaged in the first trimester with MRI
    c. can be imaged at any time provided the results will materially affect patient management
    d. can be imaged at any time following completion of satisfactory consent forms

☐ **IMAGING PROCEDURES**

Questions 9 to 11 refer to the following figure.

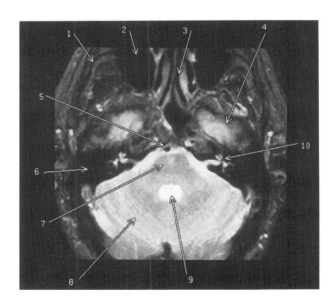

9. What type of contrast is dominant in this image?

    a. spin density   c. T2
    b. T1   d. T2*

10. Which arrow points to the internal auditory canal? _____

11. Which arrow points to the zygomatic arch? _____

Questions 12 and 13 refer to the figure below.

12. Which arrow points to the external carotid artery? _____

13. Which arrow points to the vertebral artery? _____

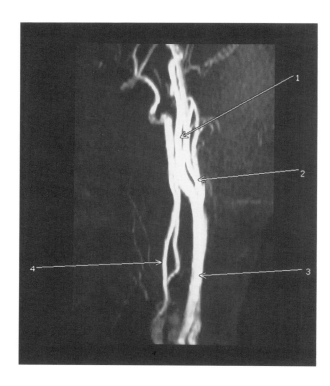

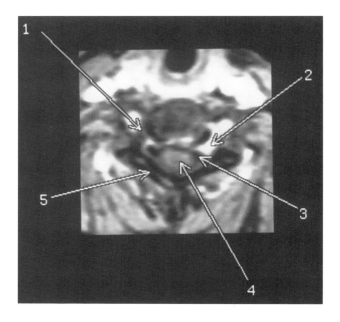

Questions 14 to 16 refer to the above figure.

14. What type of contrast is dominant in this image?

    a. spin density   c. T2
    b. T1   d. T2*

15. Which arrow points to the lamina? _____

16. Which arrow points to the subarachnoid space? _____

Questions 17 to 19 refer to the following figure.

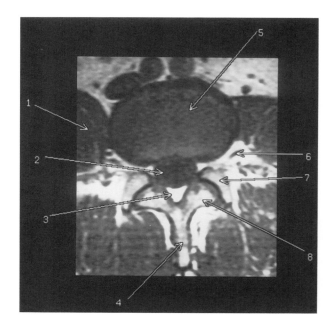

17. Which arrow points to the epidural fat? _____

18. Which arrow points to the intervertebral disc? _____

19. Which arrow points to the psoas muscle? _____

Questions 20 to 22 refer to the figure below.

20. Which arrow points to the clavicle? _____

21. Which arrow points to the liver? _____

22. Which arrow points to the right ventricle? _____

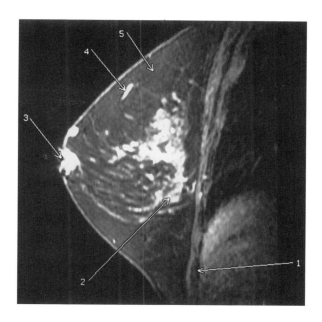

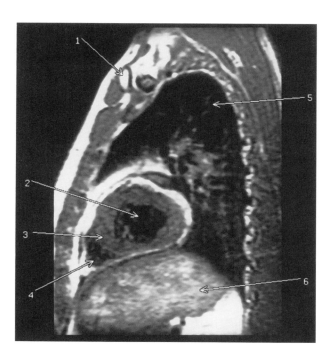

Questions 23 and 24 refer to the figure above.

23. Which arrow points to the blood vessel? _____

24. Which arrow points to the fatty tissue? _____

Questions 25 to 27 refer to the figure below.

25. What type of contrast is dominant in this image?

    a. spin density   c. T2
    b. T1   d. T2*

26. Which arrow points to the bowel? _____

27. Which arrow points to the rectum? _____

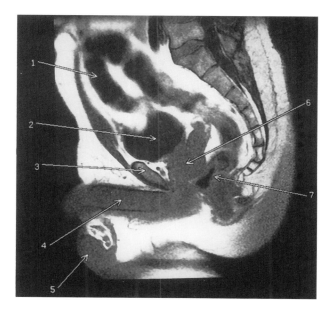

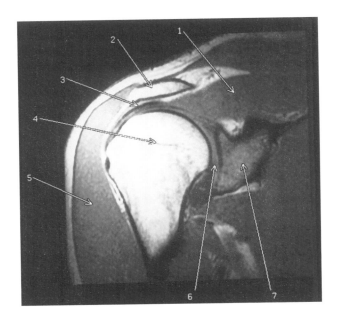

28. The structures demonstrated in this image are in what anatomical plane?

    a. transverse   c. coronal
    b. sagittal   d. oblique

29. Which arrow points to the deltoid muscle? _____

30. Which arrow points to the spraspinatus muscle? _____

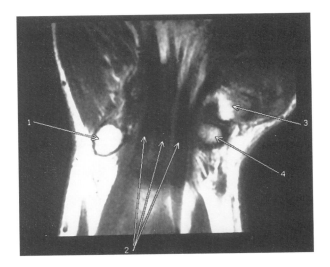

31. The structures demonstrated in this image are in what anatomical plane?

    a. transverse   c. coronal
    b. sagittal   d. oblique

32. Which arrow points to the trapezium? _____

Questions 33 and 34 refer to the figure below.

33. Which arrow points to the navicular? _____

34. Which arrow points to the subtalar joint? _____

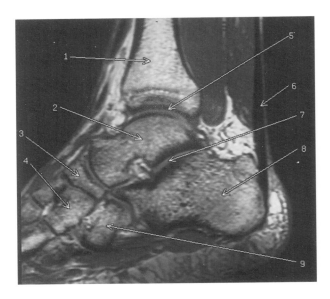

❐ DATA ACQUISITION AND PROCESSING

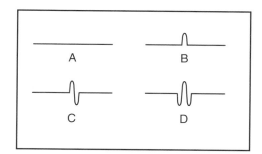

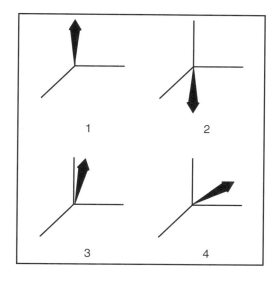

35. The symbol for a 90° RF pulse is (refer to the figure above):

    a. A   c. C
    b. B   d. D

36. Which of the following pulse sequences involves all three—TR, TE, and TI?

    a. saturation recovery
    b. inversion recovery
    c. spin echo
    d. gradient echo

37. The free induction decay is characterized as:
    (1) a constant signal for a short time
    (2) a signal decreasing in intensity
    (3) a signal increasing in intensity
    (4) a signal oscillating at the Larmor frequency

    a. 1, 2, and 3   c. 2 and 4
    b. 1 and 3   d. 4

38. A spin echo appears:

    a. immediately after a 90° RF pulse
    b. immediately after a 180° RF pulse
    c. sometime following a 90° RF pulse
    d. sometime following a 180° RF pulse

39. Match the flip angles with the appropriate vector diagram in the following figure.

    a. 0° RF _____   c. 30° RF _____
    b. 10° RF _____   d. 180° RF _____

40. In the spatial frequency domain, sharp-edged objects:

    a. contain high frequencies
    b. approach a single frequency
    c. contain a narrow range of frequencies
    d. are independent of frequency

41. Slice selection during MR imaging requires a magnetic field gradient and:

    a. a shaped RF pulse
    b. a single frequency RF pulse
    c. an inverse RF pulse
    d. a flat RF pulse

42. If a spin echo is truncated and Fourier transformed, the result appears as (see the figure below):

    a. A   c. C
    b. B   d. D

43. When a spin echo is Fourier transformed, the answer is in:

    a. Fourier space   c. Fourier frequency
    b. Fourier time   d. Fourier length

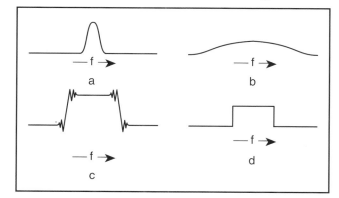

44. For a high resolution image _____ must be measured.

    a. high spin densities
    b. low spin densities
    c. high spatial frequencies
    d. low spatial frequencies

45. An entire object can be viewed as the weighted sum of:

    a. spatial frequencies
    b. temporal frequencies
    c. spin density
    d. relaxation times

46. When reconstructing an MR image, there is always a trade-off between:
(1) spatial and temporal resolution
(2) transverse and longitudinal relaxation times
(3) spatial frequencies and noise
(4) noise and spatial resolution

    a. 1, 2, and 3   c. 2 and 4
    b. 1 and 3   d. 4

47. In FSE the zero order spin echo follows the:

    a. first 180^0 RF pulse
    b. last 180^0 RF pulse
    c. weakest phase-encoding gradient pulse
    d. strongest phase-encoding gradient pulse

48. The slice select gradient is always applied:

    a. during signal detection
    b. with the phase-encoding gradient
    c. with the frequency encoding gradient
    d. at the time of the RF pulse

49. Stimulated echoes occur as a consequence of:

    a. T2 relaxation
    b. T2* relaxation
    c. equilibrium magnetization
    d. magnetization steady state

50. The two principle timing patterns in a pulse sequence diagram are:

    a. temporal resolution and contrast resolution
    b. temporal resolution and spatial resolution
    c. RF pulses and exposure time
    d. RF pulses and magnetic field gradients

51. The principle difference between an MR image and an NMR spectrometer is:

    a. B_0 intensity
    b. magnetic field gradients
    c. RF pulse sequence
    d. number of signal acquisitions

52. Slice thickness is determined by:
(1) RF pulse flip angle
(2) RF pulse bandwidth
(3) magnetic field intensity
(4) magnetic field gradient slope

    a. 1, 2, and 3   c. 2 and 4
    b. 1 and 3   d. 4

53. The effect of the pulsed phase-encoding gradient on the frequency of a column of spins is:

    a. none
    b. to increase the frequency with increasing gradient
    c. to decrease the frequency with increasing gradient
    d. to reverse the frequency

54. During the partial saturation pulse sequence the only change from one TR to the next is:

    a. the RF pulse
    b. the slice select gradient
    c. the phase-encoding gradient
    d. the frequency-encoding gradient

55. The visual receptors of the human eye include the:
(1) cornea
(2) rods
(3) pupil
(4) cones

    a. 1, 2, and 3   c. 2 and 4
    b. 1 and 3   d. all are correct

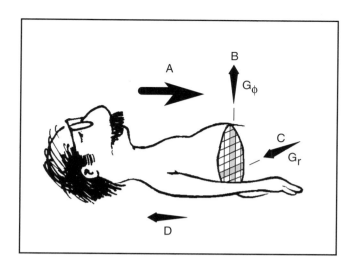

58. In a partial saturation pulse sequence, after a 90°
    RF pulse:
    (1) $M_{xy} = 0$
    (2) $M_{xy} = M_o$
    (3) $M_z = M_o$
    (4) $M_z = 0$

    a. 1, 2, and 3   c. 2 and 4
    b. 1 and 3   d. 4

59. Which tissue in the following figure has the short-
    est T2 relaxation time?

    a. A   c. C
    b. B   d. D

56. Which letter in the figure above corresponds to
    a row of spins selected by the frequency-encoding
    gradient?

    a. A   c. C
    b. B   d. D

57. At what approximate TR are the longitudinal mag-
    netization for tissues B and C equal (see the figure
    below)?

    a. 500 ms   c. 2500 ms
    b. 1500 ms   d. 3500 ms

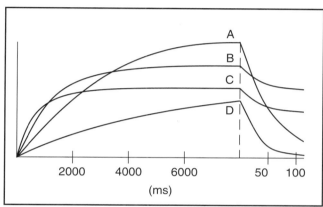

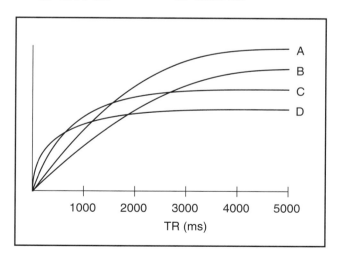

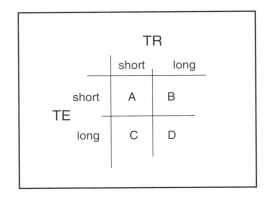

TR

		short	long
TE	short	A	B
	long	C	D

60. Which letter in the above figure represents the spin echo combination of TR and TE that results in a T2-weighted image?

   a. A   c. C
   b. B   d. D

61. For saturated spins to fully relax to equilibrium:

   a. the TE must equal the TR
   b. the TE must exceed the TR
   c. the TE must equal five T1
   d. the TR must equal five T1

62. Which of the four tissues in the following figure has the highest net magnetization at equilibrium?

   a. A   c. C
   b. B   d. D

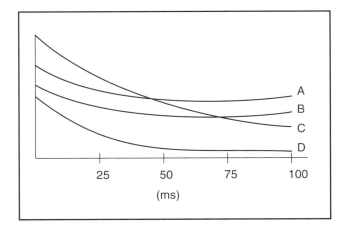

63. In a conventional spin echo pulse sequence, following the 90^0 RF pulse:
   (1) $M_{xy} = 0$
   (2) $M_{xy} = M_o$
   (3) $M_z = M_o$
   (4) $M_z = 0$

   a. 1, 2, and 3   c. 2 and 4
   b. 1 and 3   d. 4

64. The principle parameters influencing the character in an MRI pixel are:
   (1) spin density
   (2) T1 relaxation
   (3) T2 relaxation
   (4) electromagnetic induction

   a. 1, 2, and 3   c. 2 and 4
   b. 1 and 3   d. all are correct

65. The ability to detect differences in brightness level is called:

   a. contrast perception   c. color perception
   b. visual acuity   d. conspiquity

❑ PHYSICAL PRINCIPLES OF IMAGE FORMATION

66. Which of the following is **not** one of the four principle RF pulse sequences?

   a. spin echo   c. gradient echo
   b. spin gradient   d. partial saturation

67. Precession occurs when a proton spins:

   a. on the earth
   b. in a magnetic field
   c. on its axis
   d. in an electric field

68. Which of the following would be considered a discrete value, rather than a continuous value?

   a. an electric charge
   b. the electric field
   c. an electromagnetic spectrum
   d. the magnetic field

69. Power has units of:

   a. volts per second
   b. joules per second
   c. volts per coulomb
   d. joules per coulomb

70. A solenoid is a device that:

    a. has an iron core
    b. has a primary and secondary winding
    c. is a helical coil of wire
    d. is a single loop of wire

71. Electromagnetic radiation is emitted by _____ electric charges.

    a. resting   c. decelerated
    b. moving   d. compound

72. A resistive electromagnet MR imager will have the following distinct features:
(1) operation at room temperature
(2) requires cooling
(3) consists of multiple separate primary coils
(4) will contain actively shielded shim coils

    a. 1, 2, and 3   c. 2 and 4
    b. 1 and 3   d. all are correct

73. The iron yoke assembly portion of a permanent magnet imager is designed to increase:

    a. the amplitude of the magnetic field gradients
    b. the intensity of B_o
    c. the gyromagnetic ratio
    d. spin density

74. A 2 T MR imager has a field homogeneity of 5 ppm. The Larmor frequency for this imager will vary by:

    a. ± 210 Hz   c. ± 630 Hz
    b. ± 420 Hz   d. ± 840 Hz

75. Which of the following in the following figure represents a birdcage MRI RF probe?

    a. A   c. C
    b. B   d. D

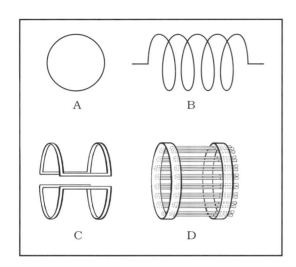

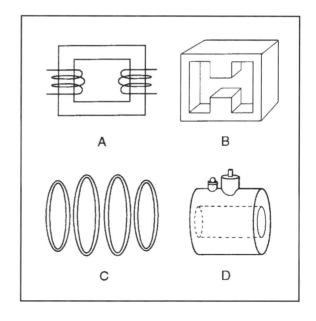

76. Which magnet in the above figure requires no electricity?

    a. A   c. C
    b. B   d. D

77. Once a superconducting imager is at field, the power required for the primary magnet coils is approximately:

    a. 0 kW   c. 20-30 kW
    b. 10-20 kW   d. 60-80 kW

78. When in the high energy state, spins are:

    a. aligned with the external magnetic field
    b. aligned against the external magnetic field
    c. spin faster
    d. spin slower

79. Net magnetization is flipped from the Z axis in order to:

    a. detect it
    b. induce spin density
    c. stimulate relaxation time
    d. measure precessional frequency

80. For a 20^0 flip angle, M_z shrinks:

    a. as much as M_{xy}
    c. more than M_{xy} grows
    b. more than M_{xy} shrinks
    d. less than M_{xy} grows

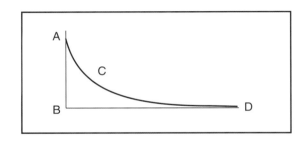

81. Spin density is most closely associated with a point at (refer to the above figure):

    a. A   c. C
    b. B   d. D

82. Transverse relaxation occurs in the _____ plane.

    a. XY   c. YZ
    b. XZ   d. oblique

83. Following a very long inversion delay time:
    (1) T1 relaxation time will be very long
    (2) T2 relaxation time will be very long
    (3) the FID will be very strong
    (4) the FID will be very weak

    a. 1, 2, and 3   c. 2 and 4
    b. 1 and 3   d. 4

84. The fluorine nucleus being investigated for in vivo NMR is:

    a. F-17   c. F-19
    b. F-18   d. F-20

85. When sampling the MRI signal, the lower limit on the sampling rate is determined by:

    a. the capacity of the computer
    b. the strength of the MRI signal
    c. the spatial frequency range of the MRI signal
    d. the rate needed to avoid aliasing

86. One line pair per millimeter is equal to _____ line pair per centimeter.

    a. 0.01   c. 1.0
    b. 0.1   d. 10

87. A useful scheme for classifying MRI artifacts would include:
    (1) magnetic field distortion artifacts
    (2) reconstruction artifacts
    (3) noise-induced artifacts
    (4) RF field distortion artifacts

    a. 1, 2, and 3   c. 2 and 4
    b. 1 and 3   d. all are correct

Appendix D

Practice Exam Answers

Exam A

1.	a	46.	b
2.	c	47.	c
3.	c	48.	d
4.	a	49.	d
5.	b	50.	c
6.	d	51.	c
7.	a	52.	c
8.	d	53.	d
9.	b	54.	a
10.	2	55.	c
11.	10	56.	b
12.	1	57.	c
13.	4	58.	d
14.	1	59.	d
15.	7	60.	a
16.	4	61.	d
17.	1	62.	d
18.	7	63.	b
19.	5	64.	b
20.	6	65.	a
21.	7	66.	d
22.	2	67.	d
23.	2	68.	c
24.	4	69.	c
25.	b	70.	d
26.	8	71.	b
27.	3	72.	b
28.	c	73.	c
29.	c	74.	a
30.	d	75.	a
31.	a	76.	c
32.	3	77.	b
33.	5	78.	b
34.	4	79.	d
35.	a	80.	b
36.	b	81.	a
37.	b	82.	d
38.	b	83.	b
39.	d	84.	d
40.	b	85.	d
41.	b	86.	a
42.	d	87.	b
43.	d		
44.	b		
45.	c		

Exam B

1.	b	46.	d
2.	c	47.	b
3.	b	48.	d
4.	b	49.	d
5.	c	50.	d
6.	b	51.	b
7.	c	52.	c
8.	c	53.	a
9.	c	54.	c
10.	10	55.	c
11.	1	56.	c
12.	2	57.	c
13.	4	58.	c
14.	b	59.	b
15.	5	60.	d
16.	3	61.	d
17.	3	62.	d
18.	6	63.	c
19.	1	64.	a
20.	1	65.	a
21.	6	66.	b
22.	4	67.	b
23.	4	68.	a
24.	5	69.	b
25.	b	70.	c
26.	1	71.	c
27.	7	72.	a
28.	c	73.	b
29.	5	74.	b
30.	1	75.	d
31.	c	76.	b
32.	3	77.	a
33.	3	78.	b
34.	7	79.	a
35.	b	80.	d
36.	b	81.	a
37.	c	82.	a
38.	d	83.	d
39.	1, 3, 4, 2	84.	c
40.	a	85.	d
41.	a	86.	d
42.	c	87.	d
43.	c		
44.	c		
45.	a		